Bionic Pioneers

JENNIFER FRENCH

and

JAMES CAVUOTO

Many of the designations used by manufacturers and sellers to distinguish their products are claimed as trademarks. Where these designations appear in the book and the authors were aware of a trademark claim, the designations have been printed with initial capital letters, for example, InterStim.

Neurotech Press
461 Second St. #124
San Francisco, CA 94107
415 546 1259
415 358 4264 (fax)
www.neurotechreports.com

For J. Thomas Mortimer
Professor, Scholar, Pioneer, and Friend

Contents

Chapter 1: Introduction

In recent years, we've witnessed enormous progress in medical technology, as researchers have devised amazing new therapies to treat debilitating diseases and disorders. The clinical researchers, investigators, and engineers who developed these new technologies have played a major role in bringing new hope to people suffering from neurological disorders who previously had few options available to them.

But this book is not about them. This book is about the real heroes who have blazed the trail to new therapies—the users of new neurotechnology products who chose to offer themselves as participants in a clinical trial or as recipients of newly approved medical devices. They have done so not only to improve their own condition, but also to advance the pace of technological progress that will undoubtedly make life even better for those that come after them.

In the chapters that follow, we will learn the life stories of 10 people with neurological conditions who made a choice to volunteer themselves for a new therapy. They will relay the often painful details of how a neurological disorder has impacted their lives. We'll examine how these users came to accept a novel or experimental neurotech therapy and take a look at how these new neurotech devices work. And

1

we'll explore how these new technologies stand to impact doctors, consumers, and researchers working in this field.

Before we begin our journey, however, it might be worthwhile to take a look at some of the neurological disorders that are affecting people today, and some of the potential neurotech therapies that have been used to treat those disorders.

What is Neurotechnology?

Neurotechnology refers to the application of electronics, or other types of signals, to the nervous system. In neurostimulation applications, electrical energy is delivered to the nervous system to achieve a therapeutic benefit. Neurostimulation devices have been used in hundreds of thousands of people to restore hearing to deaf people, reduce or eliminate chronic back pain, or restore movement to paralyzed people.

Conversely, in neurosensing applications, electronic devices record or collect signals from the brain or other parts of the nervous system. For many years, neurologists and other medical professionals have used neurosensing systems such as electroencephalography (EEG) to record brain activity and make an inference as to the mental state of an individual. More recently, neurotechnology researchers have perfected brain-computer interfaces that can record signals from individual neurons in the brain and use those signals to control a computer joystick, manipulate a robotic arm, or even restore function to a paralyzed limb.

Unlike the field of biotechnology, which explores genetic and pharmaceutical approaches to treating diseases, neurotechnology generally makes use of medical devices that are either surgically implanted within the body or used externally.

Spinal Cord Injury

It has been generally accepted that there are 300,000 individuals with spinal cord injury in the U.S., with about 10,000 new cases reported each year. Worldwide there are over 800,000 persons with spinal cord injury, with 25,000 new cases each year.

Spinal cord injury, which may involve either complete or incomplete severing of the spinal cord, almost always results in some degree of paralysis, loss of sensation, and/or impairment of internal organ function. In general, the higher the location of the injury on the spinal cord, the greater the loss of function that results. For example, patients with injury at the level of the fifth cervical vertebrae (C5) generally lose function in all four limbs (tetraplegia), while patients with injuries at the fifth thoracic vertebrae (T5) lose lower-limb function but retain the use of their upper extremities (paraplegia).

Muscle paralysis is not the only impairment of spinal cord injury. There are a host of secondary conditions that also impact the people with the condition and threaten their lives. These include the loss of sensation and sexual function, chronic neuropathic pain, pressure sores, urinary and fecal incontinence, autonomic dysreflexia, respiratory complications, as well as osteoporosis and joint contractures.

The field of functional electrical stimulation (FES), also referred to as e-stim, has emerged as one of the most promising approaches to treating and rehabilitating patients with spinal cord injury. Approximately 75 percent of people with spinal cord injury are veterans, a factor which helps explain the U.S. Department of Veterans Affairs funding support for electrical stimulation research.

After a spinal cord injury, the regions of the spinal cord

below the point of injury become isolated from the remainder of the spinal cord and the brain. Although central neural signals do not pass either to or from the areas served by the spinal cord below the point of injury, the muscles and the peripheral nerves connected to them are potentially functional. FES was developed as a means of artificially stimulating the nerves and muscles in paralyzed regions of the body so as to restore partial functionality to those regions.

Recently, researchers at the University of Louisville and UCLA have shown promising results using spinal cord stimulation in combination with physical therapy to restore voluntary movement to people paralyzed by spinal cord injury. Unlike FES, which delivers electrical stimulation directly to the paralyzed muscles, this approach attempts to reengage the spinal cord by activating dormant neural circuits that were disconnected from the brain as a result of the spinal cord injury.

Blindness

Although there has recently been some exciting progress restoring vision to blind people using retinal implants, this field is still in its infancy. In general, the human visual sense is much more complex and intricately wired than the auditory sense. Also, the amount of information that must be coded and transmitted in visual perception is much greater than in auditory perception. As a result, developing a visual prosthesis that restores significant visual function to blind people is at least several years away. Nonetheless, there are several commercial firms and research laboratories developing neural prostheses that restore some level of visual function. One approach is a retinal implant that stimulates the retina in much the same way that the cochlear implant stimulates the cochlea. Another approach involves direct stimulation of the visual cortex in the brain.

There are currently about 1.1 million legally blind individuals in the U.S. About 30 million people worldwide suffer from degenerative diseases that lead to blindness. Loss of vision impacts so many aspects of life that those of us with vision take for granted, such as the ability to drive, navigate seemlessly, or simply enjoy the colors of a sunset. Many people with visual impairments live independently but many more are dependent on care-givers, family, and friends.

The two forms of blindness that most lend themselves to a retinal implant are in patients with retinitis pigmentosa and age-related macular degeneration. Retinitis pigmentosa refers to a number of diseases that affect the photoreceptive layer of the retina. Macular degeneration refers to the loss of central vision associated with damage to the macula region of the retina.

Stroke

Stroke is currently the number three cause of death in the U.S., killing 160,000 people each year. There are 800,000 occurrences of stroke in the U.S. each year, and 4 million Americans are currently living with the effects of stroke, according to the National Stroke Association. According to the World Health Organization, approximately 15 million people suffer from a stroke each year worldwide. Of those 5 million are fatal and another 5 million are permanently disabled by a stroke.

The economic burden of stroke has been estimated at $30 billion per year in the U.S., which includes $17 billion in hospital, physician, and rehabilitation expenses, and $13 billion in indirect costs such as lost productivity.

The average cost per patient within the first 90 days after a stroke is $15,000.

A stroke is defined as an interruption of the blood flow to part of the brain. When this flow is obstructed for even a few seconds, the brain becomes starved of blood and oxygen. As a result, brain cells can die causing permanent damage. Symptoms of a stroke surface suddenly and action must be taken as quickly as possible.

There are two basic types of strokes, ischemic and hemorrhagic. Ischemic stroke occurs when a blood clot dangerously blocks arteries and stops the blood flow in the brain. Clotted strokes may happen as a result of blood vessels being clogged with the buildup of fatty deposits and cholesterol.

There are two subtypes of ischemic stroke. Embolic stroke is when a blood clot forms somewhere in the body and travels through the bloodstream into the brain. Thrombotic stroke is caused by a clot forming on a blood vessel in the brain. It grows large enough to eventually block an artery that supplied blood to the brain. Thrombosis can occur in large or small blood vessels.

Hemorrhagic stroke is a case of "bleeding" or hemorrhaging in the brain. This occurs when there is breakage in a blood vessel. There are several causes of this breakage, one being high blood pressure and another is cerebral aneurysms.

The long-term disabling effects of stroke vary depending mostly on how and in what part of the brain the stroke occurred. Typical impacts include hemiplegia (paralysis on one side of the body), impaired speech or language comprehension, impaired vision or perception, difficulty swallowing, memory loss or mood swings, and changes in emotional functioning or confusion.

Neurotechnology offers applications both in the diagnostic assessment of brain and neuromuscular damage resulting from stroke, and in therapeutic and functional electrical stimulation to rehabilitate stroke patients so they can recover lost functionality.

Parkinson's Disease and Other Movement Disorders

Movement disorders include a number of neurological disorders that affect mobility and motor functions. One of these, Parkinson's disease (PD), is characterized by selective degeneration and loss of neurons that use dopamine as a neurotransmitter from a brain area called the substantia nigra. This results in disabling motor symptoms, such as tremors, rigidity or stiffness, slowness of movements, or impaired balance and coordination. There are slow secondary symptoms that may not be as apparent but impact a person's daily function. These include loss of facial expressions, impaired fine motor dexterity, slurred speech, and loss of movement.

The symptoms of the disease not only get worse over time but can persist over a long duration. The disease progresses and intensifies at various rates; some people become severely disabled while others experience minor symptoms. As the loss of neurons continues, the chemical level of dopamine decreases and the symptoms of impaired movement and coordination worsen.

Diagnosing PD accurately has proven difficult, particularly in the early stages, as there is no proven blood or laboratory test to pinpoint a diagnosis. Physicians typically rely on medical history and a neurological examination to formulate a diagnosis. Brain scans can be performed to help exclude other diseases and disorders that mimic the symptoms of PD, such as hydrocephalus or stroke. A good response to the medication levodopa may further support a diagnosis. This medication temporarily restores the dopamine in the brain. People often seek second opinions to confirm the diagnosis.

Deep brain stimulation (DBS) has rapidly emerged as an effective treatment for the symptoms of PD after medications are no longer effective. Researchers have speculated that the changes in neuronal activity that occur with DBS may offer protection to neurons in that area and perhaps slow the progression of the disease. Recent published research suggests that the use of DBS early on in the course of the disease may help slow its progression.

Over the last several years, there have been an increasing number of research studies that point to the long-term effects of DBS in the treatment of PD.

DBS was first approved for treatment of essential tremor. Essential tremor is the most common form of tremor disorder and affects approximately 4 percent of individuals over age 40.

Dystonia, the third most common movement disorder, affects about 250,000 Americans with involuntary muscle contractions that force certain parts of the body into contorted, sometimes painful, movements or postures. Standard medical therapy, which includes oral medications and injection treatments, often proves ineffective or causes intolerable side effects. No known cure exists, although DBS has been approved for treatment of dystonia.

Urinary Incontinence

There are two main types of urinary incontinence: Urge incontinence is characterized by the frequent urge to urinate, often accompanied by leakage and discomfort. Stress incontinence results from ineffective muscle control, tissue damage, or muscle weakness within the pelvic floor. People with either form of incontinence often must wear protective devices under their clothing. Persistent incontinence can lead to embarrassing accidents, change of lifestyle, skin breakdown, and social isolation.

More than 15 million people in the U.S. suffer from urge incontinence and more than twice that number worldwide. There are currently several types of pharmaceutical products on the market used to treat urinary urge incontinence. However, these drugs have side effects such as dry mouth, dry skin, visual blurring, nausea, and constipation. The most severe cases, between 500,000 and 1.5 million individuals worldwide, are candidates for electrical stimulation treatment.

Fecal Incontinence

Fecal incontinence is the accidental passing of solid or liquid stool or mucus from the rectum. This incontinence is a signal from the body that some part of the gastrointestinal system is not working properly. The condition can be embarrassing and upsetting to people who have the condition. People often attempt to hide the problem and are ashamed to talk about it with their health care provider.

In the U.S. alone, approximately 1 in 12 adults have some form of fecal incontinence. Although it is more prevalent in older adults, it is not a sign of aging. The condition is more common among women. There are many causes for fecal incontinence, all resulting from an interference of the complex mechanisms of the muscles and nerves in and around the anal canal and rectum. Medtronic's InterStim II Therapy Device has been approved for treatment of both urinary and fecal incontinence.

Epilepsy

Epilepsy, which affects 2.3 million people in the U.S., is a neurological disorder caused by the occurrence of seizures within the brain. A seizure is typically defined as a sudden alteration of behavior due to a temporary change in electrical functioning of the brain, particularly in the outside rim called the cortex. A seizure may be minimal or very impactful, known as a grande mal. Those who experience seizures report feeling lost and exhausted, like they just ran a marathon. Severe epilepsy can lead to isolation and even prolonged hospitalization. With the proper treatment people living with epilepsy can conduct independent and fulfilling lives.

Typically epilepsy is diagnosed after the occurrence of a minimum of two seizures that are not a cause of an ancillary medical condition such as low blood pressure or withdrawal from alcohol. Physicians typically use diagnostic tools such as EEG to predict the future potential of seizures. The brain wave patterns recorded by the EEG are used not only to diagnose the condition of epilepsy but also to pinpoint the type and location of seizures. Understanding this will help the physicians prescribe a treatment method.

There are two general groups of seizures: primary and partial. Primary generalized seizures are characterized as an electrical discharge involving both sides of the brain at the same time.

Alternatively, partial seizures are initiated in a limited area of the brain. There are many different types of partial seizures depending on the person's response and area of the brain in which the electrical discharge occurs. They are typically classified into two categories: simple and complex partial seizures.

A U.S. firm called Cyberonics developed a vagus-nerve

stimulation system to treat cases of epilepsy that do not respond to other treatments such as oral medications. There are approximately 250,000 such individuals in the U.S. Other firms are investigating brain stimulation to treat epilepsy.

Amyotrophic Lateral Sclerosis

Amyotrophic lateral sclerosis (ALS), or Lou Gehrig's Disease, is a progressive neurodegenerative disease that affects nerve cells in the brain and the spinal cord. These nerve cells or motor neurons control muscle movement and organ function throughout the body. As these motor neurons deteriorate and die, it leads to paralysis, loss of organ function and eventually death of its victims. The disease gained wide recognition in the U.S. in 1939 when Lou Gehrig unexpectedly retired from professional baseball after being diagnosed with it.

ALS is a very difficult disease to diagnose and no single test or procedure is sufficient. It is through a clinical examination and series of diagnostic tests, often ruling out other diseases that mimic ALS, that a diagnosis can be established. Since it is difficult to diagnose, a second opinion is highly recommended.

The disease most commonly strikes adults between the ages of 40 and 70. ALS symptoms vary widely as well as the speed of the progression.

Muscle weakness is the most common initial symptom to surface along with frequent tripping, dropping things, abnormal fatigue of the arms and/or legs, slurred speech, twitches and/or uncontrollable periods of laughing or crying. The mean survival time with ALS is three to five years, though many people live five, 10 or more years. In a few people, the disease may remit. Not all people with ALS experience the same symptoms or the same sequences or patterns of progression. But, progressive muscle weakness and paralysis are universally experienced.

As the weakening and paralysis continue to spread to the muscles throughout the body, the victim's speech, swallowing, chewing, and breathing are eventually impaired. When the breathing muscles become affected, the person will need permanent ventilatory support in order to survive. Since ALS attacks only motor neurons, the sense of sight, touch, hearing, taste and smell are not affected. For many people, muscles of the eyes and bladder are generally not affected.

While there currently is no cure for ALS, there are some pharmaceuticals to slow the progression of the disease. There are also medical devices and therapies available to help manage the symptoms and help people maintain their independence and prolong survival.

Multiple Sclerosis

Multiple Sclerosis (MS) is a progressive immune disease attacking the central nervous system, including the brain, spinal cord, and optic nerve. The disease impacts the myelin sheath of the spinal cord. Once any part is damaged, then nerve impulses are disrupted when traveling to and from the brain or along the spinal cord. This results in a variety of symptoms of the disease.

Symptoms of MS include extreme fatigue, impaired vision, problems with balance and walking, numbness or pain, bladder and bowel symptoms, tremors, problems with memory or concentration, mood swings, or slurred speech.

The symptoms can be unpredictable and may change on a daily basis or become permanent. Symptoms are not uniform among people living with the disease. MS can be difficult to diagnose; however MRI (magnetic resonance imaging) is the best tool to detect the disease in the human nervous system.

There are four different categories of MS.

- Relapsing-Remitting is the type in which the person experiences episodes of worsening neurological function that is followed by partial or complete recovery. This is the most common type.

- Primary-Progressive is categorized by a slow progression of worsening neurological function. The progression rate varies and may include temporary plateaus.

- Secondary-Progressive is a combination of the prior two categories in which the person initially experiences a relapse-remit episode followed by a steady progression of the disease.

- Progressive-Relapsing is identified with a steady neurological decline followed by distinct relapses that may or may not result in recovery.

Rarely is MS fatal to person living with the disease. Rather, most people with MS learn to cope with the symptoms of the disease. There has been recent research and development of medications, medical devices, and exercise protocols to help people living with MS better manage the life changing symptoms.

There are a variety of neurological conditions where neurotechnology stands to benefit that are not highlighted here, such as brain injury, chronic pain, tinnitus, psychiatric disorders, and sleep apnea. We have chosen to high-light the conditions that have impacted the bionic pioneers who are profiled in the chapters that follow.

As we learn their stories, try to consider how a neuro-logical disease or disorder can impact the quality of life we have all come to cherish. Whether or not you currently suf-fer from a neurological disorder, we think it will be valuable to see how these pioneering users addressed their condi-tions and made the choices they did to explore the frontiers of medical technology.

Chapter 2: The Other Shoe Drops

The Story of Dawn Gast

It was the final straw. While on a visit to Chicago with her three youngest children ages 5, 7, and 9, Dawn tripped on a crosswalk on busy Michigan Avenue. This time she couldn't catch herself. She fell in the middle of the street and was bleeding with three young children looking down at her. "It just isn't fair," she thought. That was the final straw, when the progress of multiple sclerosis (MS) was interfering with her life as a mother.

As a busy 43-year-old full time mother of seven children and full time volunteer, Dawn didn't have time for MS to get in the way. But the symptoms were looming. She started to feel more fatigued, but what active mother of seven is not fatigued occasionally? She made excuses for the symptoms of MS, but in the back of her mind, she knew what they were. Her own mother has MS and she witnessed the signs of the disease firsthand. MS does not suddenly appear but slowly creeps into your life with initial signs of muscle weakness, reduced coordination, or blurred vision. Dawn chose to ignore the symptoms and make excuses from her busy lifestyle until she couldn't ignore it any more.

In 2005, her family made a trip to Clemson University

in South Carolina to attend a friend's graduation ceremony. While on the vacation, Dawn started to have trouble walking, had tingling in her legs, and difficulty sleeping. She stayed back in the hotel room while the family ventured out for the day. Over the course of the trip, Dawn's leg became completely immobile. "It just wasn't fair," she thought. "Here are all these great things to do as a family and I can't be there for them."

Something was wrong. Since her mother had MS, Dawn had premonitions that she might be experiencing the same thing. Back at her home in Cincinnati, OH, she did her homework on the Internet to learn about MS, mainly through the National Multiple Sclerosis Society and the Mayo Clinic. After visiting website after website, she began to think she had the disease but had to have it confirmed.

Knowing she had a family history of MS, Dawn made an appointment with her general practitioner physician. "I think I have MS," she declared to him. As a supportive doctor, he referred her to a neurologist to conduct the tests that would verify her declaration. The first neurologist did a general evaluation and simply told her to change her lifestyle and slow down. Not satisfied with that outcome, Dawn went back to her doctor for a second referral. Neurologist number two ordered an MRI but the low-quality test only monitored her brain and higher vertebrae of her spinal cord. There was nothing to confirm that she had MS. On her third referral to yet another neurologist, Dawn completed a high-quality full body MRI. From this test result, the lesions in her thoracic spinal region surfaced and finally confirmed her premonition. After six weeks of doctor's appointments, evaluations, and tests, Dawn was properly diagnosed with MS.

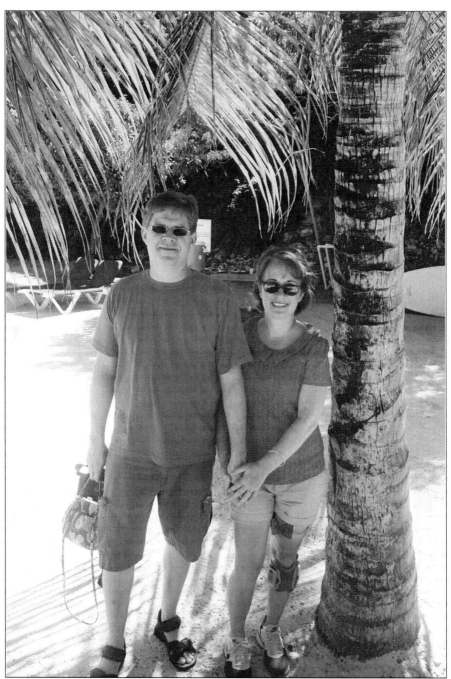

Dawn Gast wears her L300 drop foot stimulator at home and on vacation.

It was her second daughter's birthday when she received the call from her doctor. It was now reality; she had MS. Her first feeling was that it was unfair. It was unfair to her children who deserve to have an active and involved mother. It was unfair to her husband, Tony, who has to pick up the family duties where she can't. But the initial diagnosis wasn't that bad. Dawn was going into remission and the symptoms were starting to fade. At that point, it was easy for her to be in denial. Until she relapsed and the MS symptoms resurfaced, then the grief of that confirmed diagnosis came back to her. The "what if" questions started to fly around in her head. "What if I can't be at the school library" or "What if I can't pick up the kids from school?"

At first she overcame the symptoms by pure willpower. As Dawn's mobility got worse and worse, she had to compensate for her poor balance. She would hold onto the stroller or to her husband's hand. Her balance got progressively worse and she started to fall more and more. From the time she was looking up at her children on Michigan Avenue in Chicago, it was seven months after her diagnosis and Dawn knew at that point she was not safe to walk. Something needed to be done and there had to be another option.

Physical therapy might be that option. Dawn demanded a referral by her neurologist; after his reluctance, she got what she wanted—though not necessarily who. Her first physical therapist wanted to do cane training with her. He did not quite understand that a cane does not fit into her lifestyle as a mother of seven. Using a cane, she can't hold the hands of multiple children, she can't carry a cup of coffee and tend to a child, and she can't carry a lunch tray. Simple things would become difficult if not impossible. That was not the option she was seeking.

She decided to get a second opinion. Her second physical therapist took a different approach. The training he did with her focused on her lifestyle to strengthen her weak leg and learn to use this leg that she could no longer feel. After several weeks, he determined that she was not gaining any mobility improvements using compensatory strategies and it was time to look at other alternatives. He suggested that she try an external drop foot stimulation (DFS) system.

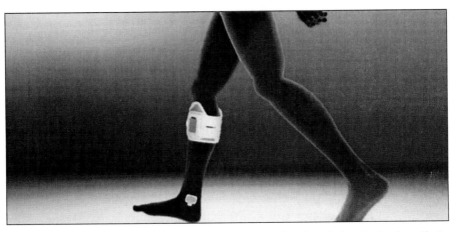

The Bioness L300 Drop Foot Stimulation system uses adaptive wireless technology that senses when a user's foot is on or off the ground and automatically adjusts to changes in walking speed and surfaces. The leg cuff produces an electrical current to activate and contract specific leg muscles. The system stimulates the appropriate nerves and muscles of the leg to override natural electrical brain signals. The system applies functional electrical stimulation in a precise sequence, which then activates the muscles to enable foot dorsiflexion and accelerate motor recovery. (Photo courtesy of Bioness Inc.)

A drop foot stimulator is a neural prosthetic worn on the outside of the body and is designed to improve the user's gait. It consists of a cuff with internal electrodes that is placed on the upper calf muscles. It also has a heel sensor placed in the shoe and a pocket control unit. Common among people living with MS or stroke survivors, drop foot syndrome is not a disease but a symptom of a condition. It is a gait abnormality in which the forefoot cannot be lifted in the stepping process as a result of muscle weakness or paralysis. Drop foot stimulation helps the user overcome this syndrome by using electrical current to stimulate the muscle. As the user attempts to lift the foot, the heel sensor activates the electrical stimulation to contract the calf muscle, lifting the forefoot. This coordinated process is controlled by the neural prosthetic to improve walking and reducing the effort in mobility.

During her next physical therapy session, Dawn's therapist obtained a Bioness L300 system for her to try. He fitted it for her leg and made a few adjustments to the stimulation.

When she tried it for the first time, "It was instantly different and I was instantly hopeful," she said. It was different because typically her leg feels like she is carrying around a big tube of sand and dragging her leg along with her. When she tried the L300, it was like "putting a stick in the sand and it made my leg feel light again." She was hopeful because her slow laborious walk turned into a productive one. For the first time in months, she felt a little less disabled. Ecstatic with this new discovery, Dawn went home from therapy to tell her husband, Tony. Appreciating this, he took off from work the next day to witness this technology in action and to understand what it was actually doing for his wife.

At that point forward, Tony was convinced that the DFS is what Dawn needed. A friend of the family hunted the internet and gathered as much information as he could find about this Bioness L300 device. When he reported his finding, it seemed too good to be true. Dawn had some doubts. But by the time they decided to get the device, Dawn was just along for the ride. Her physical therapist, her husband, and people within their support network were all supportive of her getting this new device and begin using it. But this was her doubt; "What if I relapse and I can no longer use the device?"

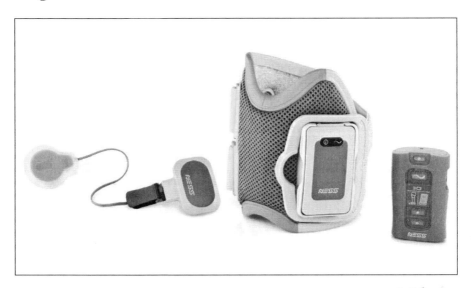

The Bioness L300 consists of three components. The leg cuff (center) is a small, light-weight device that fits just below the knee and supports consistent electrode placement for stimulation. The gait sensor (left) attaches to the shoe to detect "heel on" and "heel off" positions. It uses adaptive algorithms to communicate with the system and help patients navigate uneven surfaces, changes in elevation, and walking speeds. The hand-held remote (right) is used to turn the system on and off, select operating modes, and fine-tune settings. (Photo courtesy of Bioness Inc.)

At the time the cost of the device was equivalent to one year's worth of college tuition for one of her seven children. "That was one year of college education that my child would not receive in order for me to get this device. I feel guilty for that," she said. If she were to relapse and no longer be able to use the device, then that money would be down the drain. The doubt eventually turned to a value proposition. "What am I missing by not using the device? Is it fair to the kids to miss their activities?" Following that analysis, she became a believer and once she received the L300, there was no doubt in her mind that it was the right decision. It motivated her to work even harder.

The process of getting an L300 is not like buying a cane. It took Dawn four weeks from when she initially tried the device with her physical therapist to when she had a device of her own. First she had to convince her neurologist that she needed the L300 and to write a prescription for it. Then it was paying for the device. She submitted it to her private insurance company and the claim was denied. Not one to take no for an answer, Dawn compiled an appeal to the decision, an 18-page package including peer-reviewed published research comparing the use of an ankle-foot orthosis (a plastic brace) to the L300.

In the end, the insurance company labeled the device as experimental and denied reimbursement, even though it is approved by the FDA. The family used some money from their healthcare credit account and paid the difference out of their own pocket. Once her device was delivered, it took some time to get it calibrated properly for her body. Now affectionately called "Sparky," her L300 took several sessions to find the correct settings for how this active mom will use it. "I wanted to get the most out of this system," Dawn said.

That she did. Dawn became the active mom that she was before MS came into her life. She puts the system on when she gets dressed in the morning and it stays on until after dinner in the evening. She has the statistics to back up her performance. Without the L300, Dawn can take an average of 750 steps per day, with six stumbles per day and two falls per week. While using the L300, she can walk a mile with ease and has not fallen once while using the device.

Aside from the statistics, it is the life experiences that have had the greatest impact. For three years, Dawn's family takes an annual trip to do mission work around the world. The locations are typically poor and very inaccessible for anyone with a mobility impairment. Due to her symptoms of MS, Dawn has not been able to join her family. "I wanted to be part of something that has had a great impact on my husband and children," she said.

Once she was comfortable with her L300, she joined her family for the first time in the summer of 2012 on a trip to Bogata, Columbia. The facility where they worked had 32 steps with no railings. Her Sparky performed admirably. Over time, Dawn has been able to strengthen her muscles to the point that she can go short durations without it.

Her daughter's wedding was a special moment. Dawn did not wear the device for the entire wedding ceremony, although she put it back on for the reception. Moments like these give life to a technology that is labeled as a medical device. Considering that, what is the device really worth?

Bionic Pioneers

Chapter 3: Seizing an Opportunity

The Story of Candice Escandon

She opened her eyes and found herself on the floor of her high school chorus room flat on her back. There were Paramedics and Emergency Medical Technicians huddled around her with various medical care machines. She could see a few of her friends and her teacher who were all looking down on her. As her eyes scanned their faces, Candice wondered, "How did I get on the floor? Why does everyone look concerned? Why does my back hurt? Why am I all wet? What in the world is going on?" With that final question, she was overcome with confusion and fear.

Only a few minutes earlier, Candice, an outgoing 16-year-old, was in the hallway outside of her high school chorus room school talking with friends. She had reached for the door to the chorus room. That's when the first one hit. Candice had her first seizure.

Candice had blacked out and lost control of her bladder during the jolting of her body during the event. She ended up on the floor, feeling scared and confused. An ambulance whisked her to the local hospital to be stabilized and for some diagnostic testing. The results showed that she had had a seizure and she had hurt her back during the ordeal, but was otherwise fine. The medical team recommended that Candice consult with a neurologist. Taking the advice, her mother made an appointment but the only availability was a month later.

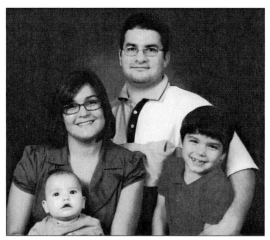

Candice Escandon and her family.

Candice's body was not going to wait a month before having more seizures. A few days later, Candice was in the backseat of her friend's car. They were driving and singing along to a song from the Backstreet Boys on the radio. She began to feel tired. The car seat began to shake. Suddenly, her friends looked back and saw Candice lying down and kicking the seat in a full seizure. When she awoke, they were in her neighbor's driveway. Candice's friends were scared, but Candice didn't understand. She sat up, looked in the mirror and began fixing her hair. Her tongue was sore.

As Candice was fixing her hair, an ambulance arrived and swept her off to the hospital and her parents would meet her there. Once at the hospital, the medical team determined that she had yet another seizure and this time she had bitten a hole through her tongue. Candice was then diagnosed with epilepsy and prescribed anti-seizure medications while she continued to wait for her appointment at the neurologist.

The incidents continued, escalating to two or three seizures per week. With each seizure, Candice landed back in the emergency room. Each time, the hospital staff consulted the scheduled neurologist who prescribed more medications. But the seizures kept coming and it became clear that waiting a few more weeks for a neurologist appointment was not an option. Less than a month after her first seizure in the chorus room, Candice was hospitalized.

As an inpatient, Candice was introduced to a new neurologist. During his initial visit, he sat next to her bed and began to talk with his young patient. Candice described her first few seizures and what she could remember. She conveyed the signals from her body that a seizure was coming, which she had learned over the past few weeks. As they talked, the doctor began to understand the situation that ignited her seizures and began to build a trust with this new client.

He concluded that there were three factors making Candice more susceptible to frequent seizures. First, prior to all of these incidents, she was going through a period of depression. Several months before, she began taking antidepressant medication to help her through this stage of her life. One of the side effects of this medication was the onset of seizure activity, originally, not a concern since Candice never had a seizure previously.

The second factor was her involvement in a car accident just a few weeks prior to ending up on the chorus floor. It was not severe but she did hit her head during the accident. The impact did not show any external signs but quietly her internal chemistry had changed.

Finally, there was family history. While in his mid-twenties, Candice's father had a series of seizures. They eventually went dormant and he never talked about it as a chronic medical condition. These three factors created a "perfect storm" in her brain, increasing her odds of experiencing seizures.

With that conclusion, the neurologist ordered an array of diagnostic tests including EEG and MRI tests. Then he gave her a difficult doctor's order; Candice was to stop going to school until her seizures could be better controlled. That news was a hard pill to swallow. Candice was a social high school student with many friends. She spent hours in the chorus room at her school and the a cappella music group was her outlet.

In a snap, she was now under a physician's care and enrolled in the hospital tutoring program. Now she was isolated from her friends and the typical American teenage life that she had known. Candice panicked about her grades, fearful that she would not be able to graduate. Her doctor explained that this was the only path to getting back to normal.

Candice began to undergo a barrage of tests and anti-seizure medications. She would take one medication and the medical team would evaluate her response. When the particular medication was unsuccessful in controlling her seizures, they would try another, then another, and another. While the litany of drug trials was difficult, Candice felt some relief that her care team was working hard to find the right combination of medications with minimal side effects to try to control her seizures.

Using an EEG, the medical team was able to find the

focal point in her brain that was causing the seizures. At that point, her neurologist described the different types of seizures and how they result from a surge of electrical activity in the brain. There are two types of seizures; primary generalized seizures, which consist of activity throughout the brain, and partial seizures, which inflict a targeted section of the brain.

The symptoms of a seizure vary from convulsions to loss of consciousness, from blurred vision to incontinence. The list is extensive and being aware of the symptoms can help people manage their condition. Candice needed to change her lifestyle to avoid triggers for her seizures. The prescription: reduce stress, no caffeine, no chocolate, and definitely no roller coasters.

Following the trial and error phase to find an effective treatment, the medical team settled on two anti-seizure medications. Unfortunately, the regimen was hardly effective for Candice. She was still experiencing multiple seizures, each happening three to four times daily and lasting about 15 minutes. The frequent seizure activity led to extreme exhaustion for Candice. She was sent home from the hospital but remained under the surveillance of her medical team, as they continued to try to find a better solution for her frequent seizure activity.

Running out of medication options, Candice's neurologist then suggested another treatment: vagus nerve stimulation (VNS) therapy. VNS therapy makes use of a surgically implanted medical device consisting of a lead electrode and a pulse generator, similar to a pacemaker. The device is implanted without brain surgery and consists of two incisions, one in the chest for the generator and one in the neck for the lead electrode. The generator is implanted in a pocket of the chest area and the lead electrode is implanted on the vagus nerve in the neck. To operate the system, the generator sends intervals of electrical stimulation to the lead electrode. The lead electrode stimulates the vagus nerve, which sends the signal to the brain. This stimulation can interrupt the "electrical storm" of seizure activity.

The system also includes a hand-held magnet, which the user or caregiver can swipe over the implant site to provide an additional dose of stimulation if there is the sensation that a seizure is coming, or while the seizure is occurring, to potentially prevent or decrease the length or severity of the seizure.

For Candice, this seemed like a promising option. For her father, it was terrifying to see his daughter undergo surgery. Candice's mother was open to the idea and wanted to learn more about the procedure and the device.

Candice's neurologist connected her family with a representative of Cyberonics, the manufacturer of the device, who thoroughly explained the technology, provided clinical research, and shared stories of other people who use the therapy on a daily basis, some positive and some not. Armed with information and a realistic perspective, Candice understood that VNS therapy works for some people but not all. She saw a ray of hope in her treatment options. If VNS therapy worked for her, she could be on the road to getting her life back, spending time with her friends and returning to singing and performing.

Yet Candice's father remained hesitant. He had concerns: the risks of surgery, having a foreign device in his daughter's body, and the potential social consequences. The family took some extra time to weigh their options. Candice's mother did some additional research regarding other treatment options and how the VNS therapy compared to those options.

Being able to afford the device was a concern but that was quickly extinguished when they found that their medical insurance would cover the device and the procedure. The family returned to the neurologist with the decision that VNS therapy was the next step. Candice agreed to have the device implanted.

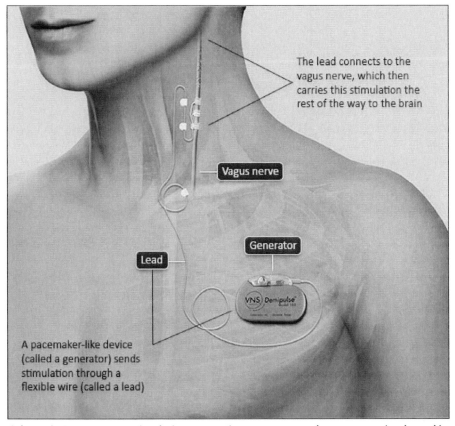

The lead connects to the vagus nerve, which then carries this stimulation the rest of the way to the brain

Vagus nerve

Generator

Lead

A pacemaker-like device (called a generator) sends stimulation through a flexible wire (called a lead)

Cyberonics' vagus nerve stimulation system incorporates a pulse generator implanted in the chest and a lead that connects to the vagus nerve. The vagus nerve connects to the brain and modulates brain and body functions. (Image courtesy of Cyberonics Inc.)

During Candice's initial consult with the neurosurgeon who would implant the device, he did not recommend the procedure for Candice. After six months of frequent seizures and hospitalizations, he believed that they had not exhausted all of her options and recommended for them to return to the neurologist for more trials for combinations of medications. After feeling like a ping-pong ball between conflicting physician recommendations, Candice returned to her neurologist, who assured them that VNS therapy was the best choice. He spoke with the neurosurgeon and advocated for VNS therapy and advised the family that he would be observing the entire procedure. Candice finally underwent the implant procedure.

One week after the surgery, Candice returned to her neurologist to have the device activated. While in his office, he connected it to the generator wirelessly and turned the stimulation system on.

With the flip of the switch, Candice could feel the stimulation and it was painful. Her body was not yet adjusted to the device and the device was not yet adjusted to her body. Altering the frequency and stimulation parameters, the neurologist sent her home. But Candice's vocal chords were impacted by the stimulation. As a singer, it was devastating. After several office visits and several adjustments to the system, they finally found the right setting for Candice to both control her seizure activity and reach a level of comfort.

A month passed and Candice began to see how her body was adapting to the device. At first, her voice would occasionally vibrate during the stimulation but that slowly subsided. Additionally, her seizure durations began to decrease. Prior to the surgery, her average seizure duration was 15 minutes. It decreased to 10 minutes and then to 7 minutes. With the decreased duration, she was able to recover more quickly from a seizure; snapping out of the seizure state within minutes rather than hours. Gradually, the frequency of her seizures also lessened from multiple times per day to a few times per week and then to one or two times per month.

With improved seizure control, Candice was able to achieve her most important goal, to return to high school in her final year and to rejoin the chorus and a cappella groups. It took some time for her to learn to use the system while she was singing. Initially, she would stop singing when she felt the stimulation begin, but eventually, she learned to sing uninterrupted with the stimulation while singing within a group.

Musical solos were different. For each solo, Candice would place the magnet over the generator and stop the stimulation. For those few minutes, she was at a greater risk of a seizure but it was not a concern for her. When she finished her solo, she would take off the magnet reactivating the system.

Slowly, life began to return to normal. The Cyberonics VNS device and her body adapted to each other and became one. Six months after the surgery, Candice began to get her independence back. With her physician's guidance, she gradually decreased the number of anti-seizure medications. Within one year post-surgery, Candice was taking only one medication. She also received a seizure alert dog to help her be aware of the onset of a seizure and to help her with the magnet if she needed it.

With her new-found independence, Candice went on to earn a bachelor's degree, marry her dedicated husband, and have two rambunctious boys who kept her busy. Her family is now enjoying the recent birth of their daughter, Eliana, who is healthy and happy. She is a, welcome addition to this close and loving family. Candice explained that she is "thankful to have the device help my brain but not be in my brain."

Cyberonics VNS therapy helped Candice gain control of her seizures, enabling her to lead a life that was more familiar to her active, social, and vibrant lifestyle. It was an option she is glad she selected.

Chapter 4: Raising His Hand to Volunteer

The Story of Jim Jatich

Pioneers are not made; they are missioned. Conventional thinking points to scientists, engineers, and entrepreneurs as the sources of innovation. They definitely have a hand in the process, but we often forget the influence that the end user, or consumer, has on the technology innovation process. Jim Jatich was one of those pioneers that shaped generations to come in neural prosthetics.

Jim was an average guy, born and raised in Northeastern Ohio. He graduated from the University of Akron with a mechanical engineering degree and went to work for Firestone in Ohio. He had a loving family and married the love of his life. He had his cherished hobbies, like playing pool, scuba diving, and working on his green Chevy Camaro. The oldest of six, Jim spent much time with his family and his younger siblings.

Unfortunately, Jim's fairy-tale marriage ended after five years and he found himself once again single. It was 1977. Jim dated here and there and found a girlfriend that he dated more frequently. Jim's brother, John, and his sister, Judy, moved into the duplex home he owned. They became

35

a tight-knit group of siblings. The home needed a fresh coat of paint, so the housemates spent a Saturday afternoon painting the house, which inevitably turned into a paint fight. Dirty, tired, and covered in paint, they decided to cool off on a warm summer's evening by taking a swim in the local lake. They grabbed some bars of soap with the intent to clean off at the same time.

Each ran off the dock to plunge into the water. First to go was John, then Judy, who looked back at Jim as he ran off the dock and dove into the cool waters. There was a pause as bubbles came to the surface. "He must be goofing off and washing his face with the soap," Judy thought. A local fisherman noticed that Jim did not resurface and notified the swimmers. Judy was the first to be near him. Now, only a few bubbles came to the surface.

When Jim dove into the lake, he hit a shallow spot, compressing his head into his spine and paralyzing him immediately. Jim couldn't move and couldn't feel a thing. Those few bubbles were from the final breath that he was able to let out of his lungs.

Being the first on the scene, Judy pulled her brother to the surface in a panic to save him. "I can't feel a thing," Jim said.

From that point on, Jim entered the world as a high quadriplegic, unable to move his four limbs, care for himself, or create the mechanical drawings that he loved to do. Life would be forever different.

Jim was taken away in an ambulance, stabilized, and placed into a rehabilitation hospital, which would become his home for the next year. The rehabilitation hospital had an institutional feel to it, with long corridors and cold walls. Jim deemed that hospital to be haunted. When his younger siblings came to visit, they felt the same thing. But his parents were dedicated to their oldest son and visited him religiously every day. Jim's dad took an early retirement from Firestone and decided to spend his time with his son.

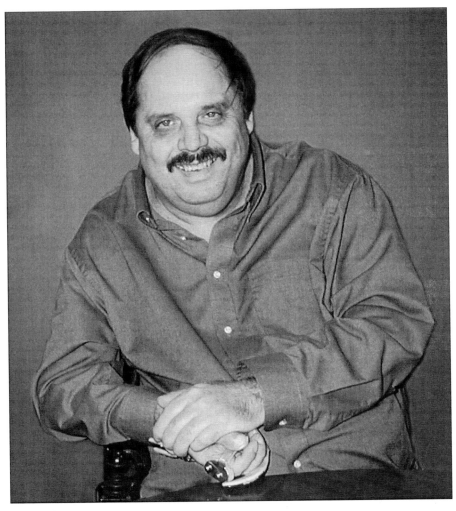

Jim Jatich

Adjusting to a life of paralysis, Jim experienced a multitude of grieving emotions. At one point, depression hit him drastically. "Mom, just go get a gun and shoot me," he exclaimed while lying motionless in his bed at the rehabilitation hospital. His mother refused to honor Jim's request as she knew he had more living to do and the Jatich family was not ready to lose the oldest son. After that episode, something clicked in Jim's mind, "I gave myself one day to feel sorry for myself. After that, I had to pick up my life and turn it around," he said. He did not know what was in store for him in the future, but Jim knew he could live with this paralysis.

It was the fall of 1978. The hot days of summer converted to the crisp air of fall in Northern Ohio. Even though Jim was a quadriplegic, he initially used a manual wheelchair. Unable to propel the wheelchair on his own, Jim would be pushed in the old Everest & Jennings wheelchair to and from his therapy appointments. It was not until years later that he would receive his first electric wheelchair and gain the ability to drive it himself.

Within those cold institutional walls, Jim was introduced to a biomedical engineer from Case Western Reserve University. Hunter Peckham was a young scientist with a warm smile and an infectious laugh. In search of a research subject, Hunter asked Jim if he would be willing to participate in some experiments using electrical stimulation of his paralyzed muscles. "I remember as if it were yesterday pushing my wheelchair down to Hunter's lab and watching him work for hours on my forearms and hands, inserting and stimulating electrodes until he controlled the right muscles," Jim recalled.

After decades of prior scientific research, electrical stimulation had been found to contract muscles that would normally be paralyzed due to a spinal cord injury. In the peripheral neuromuscular system, when electrical current is applied to a muscle, it will contract. This contraction can be designed to build an artificial nervous system restoring

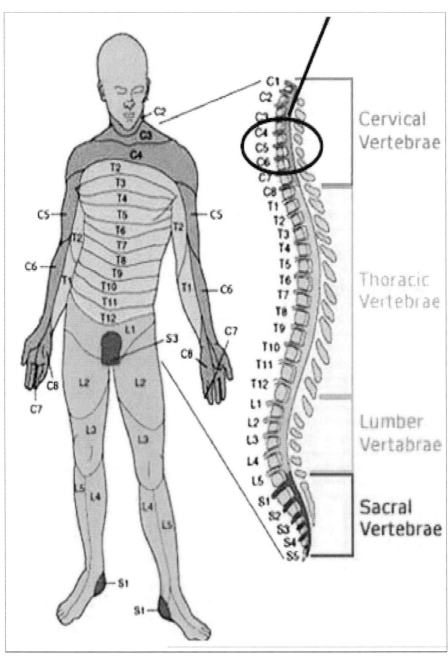

In spinal cord injury, the location of the injury on the spinal cord determines how much body function is lost. The higher the level of injury, the more function is lost. In Jim's case, his injury was at the fifth cervical vertebrae (C5), which rendered him a quadriplegic.

function to limbs that may otherwise be flaccid. Previous stimulation systems had used gel-based electrodes placed on the surface of the skin, but these systems lacked the ability to deliver stimulation precisely where it needs to go: the muscles buried deep beneath the surface of the skin. Attempting to improve on the challenges of surface stimulation, Dr. Peckham experimented with needle-like "percutaneous" electrodes that can penetrate the skin and deliver stimulation directly to the targeted muscle.

After hours of testing the placement of the electrodes, the applied stimulation was synchronized to open and close Jim's paralyzed hand. Unable to perform this simple task after his spinal cord injury, the emotion of the moment took over. "Looking down at my hand, I said, 'Wow, this thing really works! I'm actually controlling the opening and closing of my hand again.' I had just been introduced to what electrical stimulation can do to paralyzed muscles, and I was hooked."

For the next 30 years, Jim was eager to show the benefits that he gained from using electrical stimulation. Jim had found his new purpose in life and became a motivated and dedicated research participant. He was a pioneering user of Dr. Peckham's functional electrical stimulation hand system and he often traveled to scientific meetings so other researchers could see the results. The first system used the skin-penetrating percutaneous electrodes and a joystick controller. The second generation system moved the electrodes and controller inside his body after they were surgically implanted.

Being the first to volunteer, in 1986 Jim endured a nine-hour surgery for doctors to implant the electrical system into his left hand. This novel neural prosthesis restored basic hand movements. The implanted components consisted of the stimulator and eight "epimysial" electrodes placed directly on the muscle body. The stimulating electronics were placed in a pocket under the skin on the left side of the chest, similar to where a cardiac pacemaker would be located.

Seven of the electrodes were sutured to the muscles in his hand and forearm, and the wires from the electrodes were tunneled under the skin up to the left armpit, where they connected to the stimulation unit. Four electrodes controlled the movement of Jim's thumb, two others controlled the closing of the fingers, and another electrode controlled the opening of the fingers. The final electrode was a sensing electrode to help Jim control the commands of the system.

To communicate with the implanted components, a small coil was placed on the surface of the skin just over the stimulation unit. The small coil was connected to an external control unit which provided the power and controlling commands.

Jim issued input commands to the external control unit using a joystick mounted on his chest. The unit sent high-level radio frequency signals to the implanted stimulator. The implanted stimulator then decodes the messages and sends electrical stimulation to the implanted electrodes. The electrodes contracted the muscles, allowing Jim to open and close his hand.

"When I first started using the implant, I thought maybe I'd feel these wires inside and things like that. But I didn't feel anything. It didn't even feel like the implant was in there. I didn't feel any wires stretching when I moved. It was totally amazing that all of this was inside of me, with just a little external coil and a shoulder controller. It was a tremendous improvement. I could take off the shoulder controller and coil and go to the shower or swimming pool. I was astonished at how well the system worked right off the bat. And I was still amazed that I was actually controlling the opening and closing of my hand," Jim said.

Once Jim had the use of one hand, why not the second hand? Pushing the technical development of implanted neural prosthetics, the bilateral hand system now became reality. Jim underwent a second surgery to have the system implanted into his right hand. The implanted components were nearly the same as his first implanted hand system, except the new system used a combination of epimysial and intramuscular electrodes, which sat inside the muscle body.

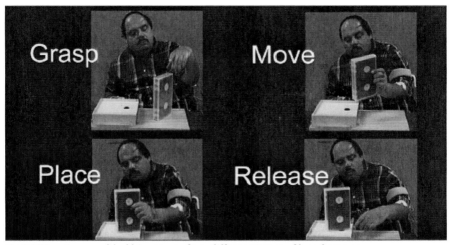

Jim's FES system enabled him to use four different types of hand grasps.

As before, seven of the eight electrodes controlled stimulated muscles to open and close the hand. However, the eighth electrode, formerly used as a sensory electrode, was now sutured to Jim's right triceps muscle. When stimulated, that eighth electrode allowed Jim to extend his elbow. The external components that he used included a shoulder controller mounted on the left side of his chest to control the right hand and a similar controller taped to his left wrist to control the left hand. By pressing the selector switch and moving his shoulder, Jim was able to open and close his hand.

As the technology progressed over the years, Jim evolved from being a research participant to becoming an integral member of the research team. In the development of electrical stimulation technology, Jim was the pioneering test pilot. A joystick taped to his shoulder sent signals to a controller implanted in his wrist. His functional hand options widened to seven different types of grasp. The coordination of stimulation for both of his hands moved to the function of both arms.

Hours in the lab testing this new system transformed to experimenting with the system in the real world. During a 1993 interview with *Scientific American Frontiers*, Jim speculated about the future input controls for this implanted electrical stimulation system. "I think the future would be maybe going towards thought control, where the person would just think, and it would just go to the implant, and you would be able to open and close your hand. That's way, way down the line. Thought control—that would be kind of neat."

Only a few years after that interview, Jim became the first research participant to test the use of brain signals recorded from the surface of his scalp as a control input for the stimulation of his paralyzed muscles.

By using electrical stimulation, Jim once again became able to perform daily actions that most people take for granted. "There are so many ways the implanted hand system has improved my life and the lives of other paralyzed people," he said. "The system's biggest benefit is the confidence and self-esteem it restores because you can use your hands again. Even the simplest of tasks, like feeding yourself in a restaurant without assistance, is a major accomplishment. Now, I am actually in control of my hand again, opening and closing it when I want. I can do things for myself."

By using the implanted hand system, Jim saw his dependency on attendant care reduce drastically. Prior to getting the system, he relied on family members and a care attendant for at least eight hours each day. For instance, they would don and doff various splints onto his paralyzed hands for eating with a fork, combing his hair with a brush, or shaving with a razor. Once he had use of the implanted hand system, Jim only needed assistance about two hours a day.

"When I get up in the morning, I do my exercises, then shower. Someone puts the system on me, which takes about five to 10 minutes, then I'm basically on my own. I only need an attendant to get me in and out of bed. My whole home and office are arranged so I can get to everything. With implants in each arm, I pick up a fork and feed myself, pick up a pen and write, and type on the computer. I no longer rely on straws or people giving me drinks anymore: I can simply pick up a glass and drink."

Once Jim got up and into his power wheelchair, he became independent through his home and also outside his home. He even gained the independence to be home alone without a caregiver.

Jim complimented the system for giving time back to his father and other family members that they would otherwise use to help him. "And it has given me a greater sense of independence," he declared. The system gave him control of his life. "I benefitted immensely from being able to extend my elbow. I could add 'weight shifts' to relieve pressure on my body from sitting in my wheelchair for a long time. Using elbow extension alone in both arms I could partially push a manual wheelchair."

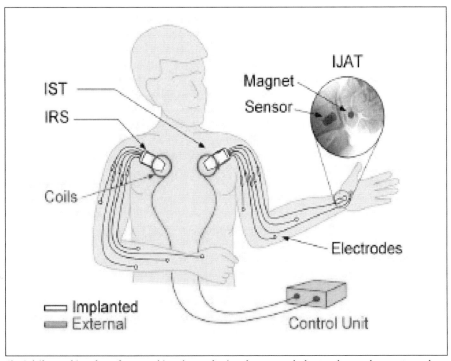

Jim's bilateral implant featured implanted stimulators and electrodes and an external control unit electromagnetic coils positioned over the stimulators on each side of his body. (Image courtesy of Cleveland FES Center)

Jim dedicated three decades to electrical stimulation research. He was a member of the research team; advocating in Congress, speaking with the Vice President, Surgeon General, and generations of NIH program managers. Jim advised the FES Center on policy development, research funding, clinician training, and public relations. He was energized by helping others with spinal cord injuries. When he would see someone else using their hands with the implanted system, it made him happy. "I smile at how motivated they are to face life's challenges. It's worth all the surgeries and electrodes in my hand, all the pain that we've gone through and all the research and development." This reflection by Jim shows how he made neural prosthesis research his new purpose in life.

"I feel that what we have accomplished so far is a great step toward independence for spinal cord injured people. I guess that's what has kept me going with the program. It also brought me joy to see the results. I know how this has changed my life, and I wanted the same feeling for every other spinal cord injury patient."

This pioneer of implanted neural prosthetics used his system actively for over 30 years. Jim Jatich passed away peacefully on September 6, 2013 due to complications of secondary conditions from his spinal cord injury. Jim was a great fighter and role model to many.

Chapter 5: A Mom's Second Look

The Story of Kim O'Shea

W e've all heard the expression, "You don't value something until you lose it." For Kim O'Shea, that expression has a profound meaning. When she was 12 years old Kim was diagnosed with retinitis pigmentosa, a degenerative disease that leads to blindness. She also has macular edema which accelerates the progression of retinitis pigmentosa. By the time she was 28, she had lost 80 percent of her vision and was registered as legally blind.

Two years later, at age 30, Kim and her husband, Sean, celebrated the birth of their second daughter. But it was a difficult time for Kim. Aside from postpartum depression, she was grieving the loss of her own vision, which by then was only tunnel vision.

It's never an easy task caring for two small children but doing so when visually impaired is even more challenging. Kim began to rely more on her husband to help with the parenting duties. It was difficult for Kim not to be able to do what other moms do with their children.

Then one day while listening to the news, Kim learned of a new technology that could restore vision to blind people.

At the time, Second Sight Medical Products, a California-based neurotechnology startup firm, was conducting a clinical trial of its Argus II retinal prosthesis. Although the system was new and experimental Kim thought that she had nothing to lose by exploring it.

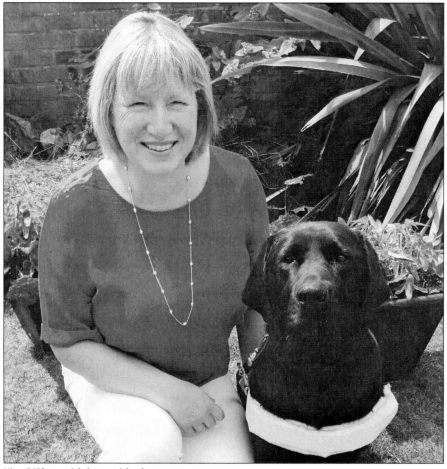

Kim O'Shea with her guide dog.

The Argus II retinal implant is surgically implanted in the user's eye. It consists of a pair of glasses, a cable, and a video processing unit. There is also a surgically implanted electrode array and antenna that are placed on the retina of the user. A small video camera attached to the eyeglasses sends images to the video processing unit, which then transmits wirelessly to an implanted electrode array in the retina. The electrode array currently has 60 elements. These elements bypass the damaged photoreceptors in the retina and directly stimulate neurons that lead into the optic nerve. The user learns to interpret the signals as visual images.

Before she could be selected as a participant in the clinical trial, Kim had to undergo many hours of testing, including a psychological test. She passed those tests but was still uncertain whether to undergo the implant procedure. Her primary concern was the commitment of time it would take. Time to go to and from the hospital once or twice each week. Time to partake in a surgical procedure and recovery. Time to learn the new system, endure hours of testing and complete the homework when it was assigned.

Kim's family would need to sign on to this; if they did not support her then there was no point in her participating. After discussing it at length, the family decided there was everything to gain and nothing to lose. Kim and Sean made a point of managing their expectations. They knew it would be a long and slow process and it was difficult to predict how much, if any, visual function she would recover. Kim's daughters graciously encouraged her. "Mum, just go do it," they advised. Appreciating her family's involvement, Kim became excited for a new beginning and a new challenge. Fortunately, all the costs associated with the system and the surgery were paid for by the clinical study.

In August of 2009 Kim underwent the implantation surgery for the Argus II. The surgery took four hours and it took a couple weeks for her to recover from the surgery.

Once she was ready for testing, the research team working with Kim turned the system on. A member of the team instructed Kim to look toward the hallway. At first she saw nothing. But when she turned her head she saw a spark of light. "Oh my gosh!" she exclaimed. Over time, working with the new system, Kim would be able to discern letters, numbers, and shapes as she learned how to use her now retinal implant system.

Kim spent many hours with the research team who performed experiments in the lab that required her to repeat common tasks like identifying shapes. Once she progressed, Kim took the system home, spending time learning to see letters, numbers, and shapes. She also tested the system in the outside world, using it to walk a defined path to see if she could differentiate between the pedestrian walkway and the street.

Kim doesn't use the system as much while at home simply because she knows where everything is in her house and she finds it quicker to get things done without the system. But when she's outside the home Kim uses the system to detect movement of people or cars nearby. She is pleased that she's able to identify her husband's face out of a crowd of people. She also appreciates being able to see her pets move around in her back yard. Her one complaint is that she would prefer a choice of glasses to fit her personal fashion style.

One day the research team was testing her perception of color. They tweaked one of the stimulating electrodes and Kim found that she could see the color blue. "Oh my, that is blue!" Kim shouted. She had not seen any color for many years and this was an amazing development for her. Although the research team wanted to test other colors, Kim kept asking to see the color blue again.

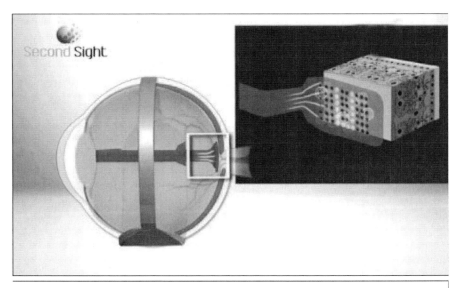

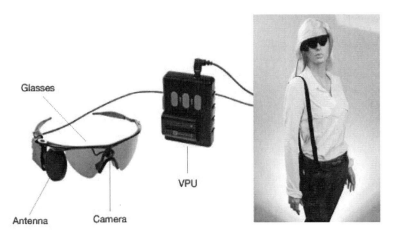

The Argus II retinal implant system from Second Sight features an electrode array surgically implanted in the eye, an electronic case, and an antenna. The external equipment includes glasses, a video camera, a video processing unit (VPU), and a cable. Video signals from the camera are sent to the VPU, processed, and transformed into instructions that are sent back to the glasses via a cable. These instructions are transmitted wirelessly to the antenna in the implant. The signals are then sent to the 60-element electrode array, which emits small pulses of electricity. These pulses are intended to bypass the damaged photoreceptors and stimulate the retina's remaining cells, which transmit the visual information along the optic nerve to the brain. This process is intended to create the perception of patterns of light which users learn to interpret as visual patterns. (Images courtesy of Second Sight Medical Products Inc.)

Prior to this experiment, Kim was only able to see shades gray. The addition of color to the system allowed her to perceive her environment in a three-dimensional manner.

As a pioneering user, Kim has been providing valuable feedback to the research team on how consumers use the system. She believes that the use of color can help provide depth perception. Input that she provides helps to improve the next generation of this technology. She still relies on her guide dog for independence but she looks forward to the day when she can get around without additional aids.

Chapter 6: Stimulation Lends a Hand

The Story of Andrew Genge

A ndrew Genge was a healthy 15 year-old playing for his high school rugby team in Oshawa, Ontario. In a hard-fought game Andrew executed a big tackle on a player from the other team. In the maneuver, his opponent's hipbone collided with Andrew's face, breaking his jawbone, slicing into his carotid artery, and sending a blood clot to his brain.

It was three in the afternoon and Andrew was rushed to emergency services. He was stabilized and treated for his apparent injuries but the blood clot went undetected. Four hours after the accident, he started to feel the symptoms of a stroke. His right arm became weak. When he tried to speak to alert the medical personnel, he could only produce a few grunts and no comprehensive words. Reasoning that it was a side effect of the pain medications, Andrew went to sleep. At midnight, the blood clot released, damaging sections of Andrew's brain and leaving him with paralysis on the right side of his body. This athletic high school student was now unable to move or speak as freely as he once did just 24 hours earlier.

His first memory after that evening was when he awoke

in the intensive care unit. A high school friend was visiting him. Andrew recognized him and attempted to say "Hello," but he was not able to speak. In addition to the paralysis, the stroke impacted Andrew's speech capacities. For the first six months, he could make utterances but not form comprehensive words or sentences. After working with a speech therapist for nearly one year, he regained the ability to speak.

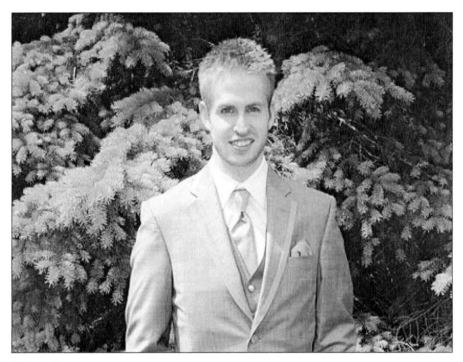

Andrew Genge

Along with speech therapy, physical and occupational therapies were included in Andrew's rehabilitation process. Undergoing conventional methods of stroke therapy, he slowly progressed during the first year but began to plateau after 18 months. While reading the newspaper, Andrew's mother learned of a research study recruiting stroke survivors for an experimental electrical stimulation therapy. Intrigued by the article, she did her own research about the study. Taking the potential risks and the time commitment into consideration, she concluded it might be a good possibility for her son.

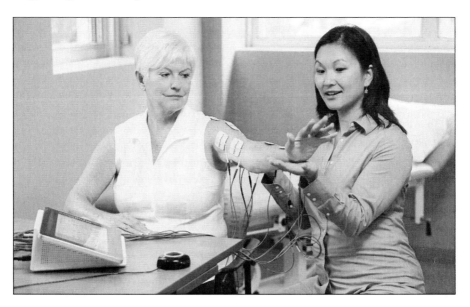

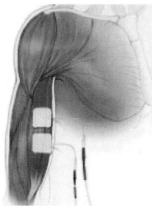

The MyndMove system, developed at Toronto Rehab and the University of Toronto, uses embedded stimulation protocols that can elicit more than 30 different reaching and grasping movements in people with upper-limb paralysis. It includes an eight-channel stimulator that can stimulate up to eight different muscle groups. Each protocol specifies the sequence of muscle stimulation required to precipitate a natural movement and practice a functional task. During therapy, patients participate by actively attempting the desired movements. Therapists guide the timing and quality of the desired movements and the MyndMove device delivers stimulation to elicit the movements. (Photo courtesy of MyndTec Inc.)

Andrew and his mother took the one-hour drive to the Toronto Rehabilitation Institute so he could be tested as a candidate. Although he responded to the tests and proved he was a good candidate, the trial was several weeks from launching. In the meantime, the investigator referred Andrew for physical therapy sessions.

The call finally came. The research team was executing the study and extended an invitation to Andrew for his initial visit. That first visit was focused on collecting baseline data. Andrew completed various tasks using only his weak right arm and hand, without any assistance.

Upon his first introduction to the functional electrical stimulation device, Andrew thought, "This is a weird contraption." The programmable electrical stimulator offered the ability to customize stimulation patterns for various applications. External gel-coated electrodes and a small external controller produced the transcutaneous electrical stimulation.

The electrodes are strategically placed on the surface of the skin, for example on the forearm between the wrist and the elbow. Participants are challenged to perform various repetitive motion tasks using their paralyzed hand while the device delivers electrical stimulation through the electrodes. The stimulation activates muscles in the forearm to contract with the desired motion. The sessions last an hour and continue five days per week for a minimum of three weeks.

When the research team placed the electrodes on Andrew's arm and turned the system on he responded immediately. "Wow! My arm is moving," he exclaimed. He felt a tingling sensation with the stimulation but his focus was on the movement of his paralyzed hand.

For six months, Andrew and his mother drove to the laboratory for Andrew to receive the electrical stimulation therapy. He began to see the benefits of the sessions. He gained the ability to open and close his hand--even without the stimulation--as well as extend his fingers. Six months turned into two years of therapy. Andrew now experiences the functional improvement at home. He can perform activities of daily living, such as loading the dishwasher and using a keyboard, much faster while using his once-paralyzed right hand.

It has been overwhelming for Andres to get the use of his right arm back. Even though therapy has stopped, he continues to go to the gym and exercise his right side, the side impacted by the stroke. Andrew describes himself as an optimist with a goal to regain all of his capacities. Nine years after that big tackle, he has almost full function in his right side. He is working at the local Abilities Center and going to school to become a therapist himself.

Bionic Pioneers

Chapter 7: The Rebirth of Normalcy

The Story of Lauren Henderberg

"This too shall pass." We often tell ourselves this when we have an ache or a bodily complication that is out of the ordinary. For Lauren, it was a matter of getting her body back to normal after giving birth to her first daughter, Evelyn.

Craig, her husband, and Lauren were anxiously awaiting the birth of their first child. That moment did not come until almost two weeks past her due date, when they agreed to induce labor.

Inducing did not make the process any quicker. Lauren went into the hospital on Monday and did not deliver their daughter until Wednesday. During the birthing process, they found the baby in an occiput posterior position in which the back of the baby's head presses against the mother's tailbone and the baby is face down going through the birth canal, also known as sunny-side up. After three hours of pushing, the physician used a set of forceps to help pull the baby out. Those forceps would become Lauren's nemesis and set in motion a long and arduous condition that Lauren would endure for several years.

While using the forceps for the delivery, Lauren's skin

was torn—a third degree tear. She briefly dislocated her hip and suffered severe hemorrhaging. All of this resulted in fecal incontinence. Regardless of her condition, Lauren and Craig were thrilled to have a healthy, new baby girl. By Friday, two days after the birth, Lauren and baby Evelyn were released from the hospital. With a dislocated hip, bruising, many stitches, and incontinence, Lauren thought, "All of this will resolve in a matter of time." Being a happy new mother, she accepted her condition as a matter of consequence.

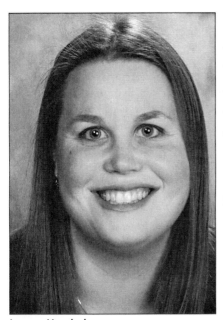

Lauren Henderberg

It is typical for women after giving childbirth, for their bowel and bladder functions to take some time to return to normal. It was about two weeks after the delivery when Lauren had her first bowel movement, but that was not normal. She could feel the discharge running down her leg with no other indications. She had no control over it, no sensation. There was just a disconnect between her brain and her bowels.

This too shall pass, right? Here is Lauren, a new mother with her own physical recovery and incontinence. Now, Baby Evelyn developed infant colic, crying for long periods of time during the day and night. Lauren was stressed, tired, and sore.

Still, for Lauren, this seemed normal. She was aware that all new mothers go through a difficult transition and this situation was no different from what mothers have experienced for decades. She kept telling herself, "This will pass."

It wasn't until she had a six-week follow-up exam with her doctor did Lauren suspect that the incontinence was not a "typical" experience of a post-partum mother. The doctor with whom she had her appointment was also the doctor who used the forceps for the delivery of her daughter. During her follow-up appointment, the doctor did a rectal exam on Lauren and told her to squeeze her rectum. Lauren thought she was following the instructions but there was no force. Again, the doctor said, "Squeeze." Lauren replied, "I am," but there was still nothing. After the exam, the doctor reassured Lauren that having bowel incontinence was normal after giving birth and she should not worry about the condition, as it will resolve itself as the body heals.

Lauren went back home to deal with the fecal incontinence condition that seemed to persist. The incontinence continued and her repertoire of embarrassing moments started to build. Once, she was at a park with her husband and Evelyn. Lauren thought she just simply passed gas, but she ended up having fecal incontinence too. She ran to a restroom to clean herself up. On another occasion, she was driving to a friend's house for a play day with the children and had an accident in the car. Lauren found herself driving to the store instead to purchase underwear since the incontinence damaged her current pair beyond repair.

Being out in public and having a bowel accident was embarrassing. With each embarrassing moment, Lauren started to change her behavior. She started carrying her own diaper bag along with the bag for her daughter. Her bag contained an extra pair of underwear, clothing, incontinence protection, and cleaning supplies. She would keep extra clothes and supplies in her car and in her closet at work. Everywhere she went, she had to be prepared for a fecal incontinence accident. She began to pull back on activities outside of her home and refrained from going anywhere that was a distance from a restroom or porto-let. Lauren even stopped her walks around the neighborhood for fear of having yet another accident with no place to go. Gradually, she found herself staying at home, unable to leave.

The incontinence not only took a toll on Lauren's physical health and lifestyle but also on her mental health. Daily accidents, daily embarrassment, daily setbacks began to wear on Lauren emotionally. She began having nightmares, which turned into insomnia. At the time, it did not seem outrageously unusual since most new mothers have little sleep. But the insomnia morphed into high levels of anxiety, then escalating into panic attacks. They came with triggers. The fecal incontinence was a trigger for her. With each accident, Lauren would have a panic attack. Another common trigger was hearing two forks hit each other, which reminded her of the forceps from the delivery. She would be at a restaurant, hear that sound and find herself huddled under the table in a panic. There was simply no way to control when and where the panic attacks would occur.

Over a six-month period, these incidents started to escalate to a point where they impacted her well-being and she began to have symptoms of post traumatic stress disorder. Later, she confided in her great uncle, a retired OB-GYN and gynecologist. She described her situation and the frequent incontinence that she was experiencing. "That is *not* normal," he advised her and recommended she get a second opinion. After six months of dealing with this condition, she found a new doctor.

She also sought out a mental health professional to help her with the panic attacks that she was experiencing. At that point, Lauren wanted to make it clear that she was not experiencing post-partum depression. The treatments for postpartum depression and post traumatic stress disorder (PTSD) are very different. She wanted to make it clear that depression was not part of her symptoms; anxiety was a large component of her symptoms.

Her first psychologist did issue a diagnosis of high anxiety and then PTSD. The recommended treatment was a cognitive behavioral approach, which involves talking through the triggers that Lauren was experiencing. But Lauren needed to process what was happening to her--not simply talk about it.

Still experiencing her PTSD symptoms, Lauren reached out to a second psychologist who recommended a therapy specifically targeted for the treatment of trauma, Eye Movement Desensitization and Reprocessing (EMDR) therapy. This is a three-stage treatment with a goal of understanding and gaining a perspective on emotions that lead to healthy and useful behaviors. This therapy was coupled with oversight by a psychiatrist, who prescribed targeted pharmaceuticals rather than a blanket anti-anxiety medication.

Throughout these treatments, Lauren remained isolated. This is not how she had envisioned it would be as a new mother. She decided that she and Craig were not going to have a second child because of the trauma she experienced with the first delivery.

Lauren made an appointment with a gastroenterologist physician and then with a rectal surgeon. It was finally determined that Lauren had a tear of her perineum, the skin between the vagina and the anus, which caused a defect in her rectal sphincter. Once diagnosed, she began targeted physical therapy to attempt to strengthen the muscles.

The first treatment in her physical therapy was the use of a vaginal probe for biofeedback therapy in which the probe is used with various exercises to help to improve muscle strength in the pelvic floor. This therapy helped a little but because it was a vaginal probe it did not have an accurate gauge on the strength of her pelvic floor and sphincter muscles. After receiving this treatment for several months, Lauren turned to a women's health specialist for physical therapy.

With this new physical therapist, Lauren began scar reduction therapy. Since her perineum was completely torn during childbirth, the skin began to heal on its own. As that skin healed, it pulled the sphincter open, which was a large contributor to her incontinence. The therapy was focused on reducing the pulling effect from the scar tissue.

The new physical therapist started trigger point therapy in the rectal area using biofeedback. Lauren also learned some exercises to perform in order to help strengthen the pelvic floor and abdominal muscles in the area presumed to be weakened by childbirth. These exercises helped Lauren to compensate for her weak rectal sphincter but did not solve the incontinence problem she continued to experience. For three years, Lauren endured physical therapy for these muscles. It was helping her condition a little but not solving it, but there was no other alternative. Lauren's choice was to continue to exercise or do nothing at all.

During those three years, Lauren continued to pull back on activities outside of her home. Lauren went back to work as a special needs teacher the following fall, six months after Evelyn's birth, despite the incontinence. Every day Lauren would have at least one accident at work. She would need to wear protection and sometimes leave the classroom to change her soiled clothes. She endured this for the entire school year. She went back the following September until one day in the late spring. Lauren had a fecal incontinence accident accompanied by a panic attack that landed her in the hospital. That was the breaking point. Lauren could no longer be a teacher, a profession that she loved.

Lauren's rectal surgeon kept encouraging her to continue with physical therapy. For those three years, the surgeon informed Lauren of the other surgical options but did not recommend them for her specific condition. One option was for reconstructive surgery of the sphincter, but it would need to be performed every five years. The doctor did not want Lauren, a young woman of child-bearing age, to experience such trauma to her body. Her surgeon was hopeful for a new therapy that was going through the approval process.

The day finally came when Lauren was introduced to the InterStim II Therapy Device. "This is what you have been waiting for," said Lauren's rectal surgeon. "You are a perfect candidate for it." The InterStim II system is a surgically implanted device used to send mild electrical pulses to the sacral nerves and designed to treat overactive bladder, urinary retention, fecal incontinence, and constipation. It consists of three components. The implantable neurostimulator is placed under the skin and in the lower abdomen or back region. The electrodes are thin wires that carry electrical pulses to the nerves controlling the pelvic floor. Finally, there is a hand-held remote as a programming tool used to adjust the strength of the stimulation and to turn it on and off. A trial device is initially implanted to gauge whether or not the patient will respond to the therapy. If successful, then a permanent system is implanted in place of the temporary one.

With that first introduction, Lauren thought, "This is awesome." She followed that reaction with, "You are going to put what in my body?" Regardless, she was attracted to the fact that there would be no major incisions, no more surgeries on the sphincter, no more invasive work to the area damaged by the forceps.

Despite her enthusiasm from her introduction, Lauren wanted to do her research to learn more about this new treatment. At the time, the InterStim II Therapy device had been recently approved by the FDA for fecal incontinence, so the only patient history available was that from the prior clinical trials. However, the InterStim II Therapy Device used for bladder incontinence had a long clinical history and Lauren drew from that to help gain knowledge about the procedure and what to expect.

Lauren and Craig discussed this new option for her long-standing condition, along with the risks and benefits. Lauren had endured physical therapy for three years and was excited there was something new to try. They liked the fact that there would be no more cutting of her sphincter.

Once they saw the success of others who were in the clinical trial, it was hard for Lauren and Craig to curb their enthusiasm. Still, there were real risks to consider. If Lauren was implanted with this device, she would never be able to get an MRI. If they ever decided to have another baby, it was unclear whether or not the use of the device would be safe for the developing unborn child. Finally, what would they do if it didn't work? Lauren had been through enough trauma and was making progress with her therapy; a failed surgery might be devastating for her.

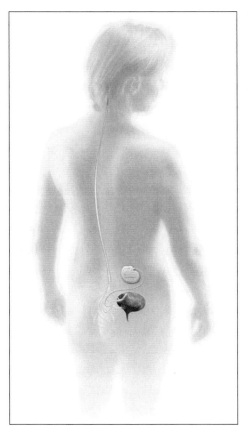

The implantable InterStim system uses mild electrical stimulation of the sacral nerves to influence the behavior of the pelvic floor muscles and bowel. InterStim therapy uses an implantable system, consisting of a thin wire lead and a neurostimulator, or pacemaker-like device, as well as external clinician and patient programmers. (Image courtesy of Medtronic Inc.)

The biggest concern for Craig and Lauren was the financial burden. They had gone from a dual income household to a single income family. They considered themselves to be prudent savers. Prior to the birth of Evelyn, Craig and Lauren built a nice nest-egg for the newborn addition to their family. But that nest-egg was depleted by medical bills— out-of-pocket costs for physical therapy, EMDR therapy, medications, copayments for the rectal surgeon, and hospital visits resulting from her panic attacks. All of these expenses drew down any savings they had. How would they pay for a new medical device along with the implantation surgery? What if the insurance wouldn't cover it? Where would they get the money? Sell a car? Take out a loan?

Initially, their health insurance denied coverage for Lauren to get the InterStim II Therapy Device. Following an appeal, their insurer eventually approved coverage with standard copayments.

With insurance approval in hand, Lauren proceeded with the two-week trial period for the device. This was an outpatient surgery to implant a temporary device. A few days after the surgery, Lauren began to notice a difference. "It was like my brain was connected to my sphincter again." Her fecal incontinence accidents significantly reduced. Excited to learn that the trial was successful, Lauren could not wait to get the permanently implanted device.

On August 5, 2011, Lauren gave her surgeon a big hug prior to getting the InterStim II Therapy Device permanently implanted. Prior to going home from the hospital, the medical team tuned the system to Lauren's specific body needs. When they first turned it on Lauren said it felt weird. She had had no sensation in the pelvic floor in three years and now she felt the stimulation. There were a few jolts of stimulation while they were tuning the system but not for long.

Her recovery from the surgery took approximately one month while her family and friends helped her around the home and with the care of Evelyn. Lauren started to be active again, walking the neighborhood and doing pool therapy. All in all, she was getting her life back together. She was released from both physical and psychological therapy. Even the financial burden of all the additional medical expenses started to subside. During her three-year fight with incontinence, Lauren felt like she had her life back. Craig and Lauren breathed a collective sigh of relief.

At the same time, Craig and Lauren began to explore the possibility of a second child. Three years prior, Lauren was convinced that she would not have another child, especially after her first experience. They always wanted more children but the previous circumstances and Lauren's chronic condition stripped them of that dream. Now that Lauren was able to exercise, be social, and have a normal life, it was a real possibility again.

Her rectal surgeon and OB-GYN worked together as a team to help Lauren. For the safety of the baby, Lauren would need to turn the device off during the nine-month pregnancy, which brought the return of her fecal incontinence. Lauren also developed complications and was placed on bed-rest at 20 weeks.

She gave birth to a healthy baby boy, Elliott, via elective C-section procedure, returned home and eagerly turned the InterStim II Therapy Device back on to alleviate her incontinence symptoms.

Lauren emerged from this experience as an advocate. She had wished she had another user to talk to while making her decision about the InterStim II Therapy Device. She is now available for others who might want her advice. Following her implantation surgery in August 2011, Lauren started a blog, mainly to keep family and friends updated and express the circumstances around her incontinence. Later that blog became an advisory tool to tell others about her experience, let them know that they are not alone, and to seek treatment rather than tolerate an isolating life of incontinence. During her three-year journey, Lauren found it very difficult getting access to the right medical care professionals. Her final team was fantastic, but it took a long time to assemble them. Lauren later joined the volunteer ambassador program with Medtronic for fecal incontinence.

One year after receiving the InterStim II Therapy Device, Lauren and Craig hosted an Anniversary Party, later named the "Assiversary Party," inviting friends and family over to their house to share how Lauren's life had changed for the better. Going from isolation to the relief of getting her quality of life back was worthy of a time of celebration.

Chapter 8: A Breath of Fresh Air

The Story of Matt June

It is all too common for neurotechnology devices to be an option of last resort. It is a precarious situation in which all other options have been attempted with no success. In this particular situation, Matt June bucks the trend. This is the story of one family using technology to stay two steps ahead of the progressive condition of Lou Gehrig's disease or ALS. This is also a story about maintaining quality of life. Quality of life is often talked about but it's hard to describe exactly what it means. Each individual defines it differently. The impact of quality of life is not always realized until it is compromised.

After serving four years in the U.S. Army, Matt June returned to his home in the small rural town of Steubenville, OH and took a job with the U.S. Postal Service. For years, Matt was a clerk in the offices but eventually he became a carrier with his own route. This 41 year-old father of five had a pretty "normal" American life. The first time he suspected something was not quite right was when he was trimming his fingernails and had difficulty putting pressure on the clippers. Then he started to have trouble gripping a baseball and running between the bases. It was like

71

something was seeping into his life, but he did not know what.

It wasn't until Matt started falling and those falls began interfering with his carrier route that he decided to see his doctor. Matt was referred to a rheumatologist who suspected that he had myositis, an inflammation of the muscles that causes weakness and fatigue. Not fully satisfied with the diagnosis matching his observed symptoms, Matt sought another opinion, this time from a neurologist. It was September 2009 when he confirmed the diagnosis. It was not myositis but a more progressive condition of ALS.

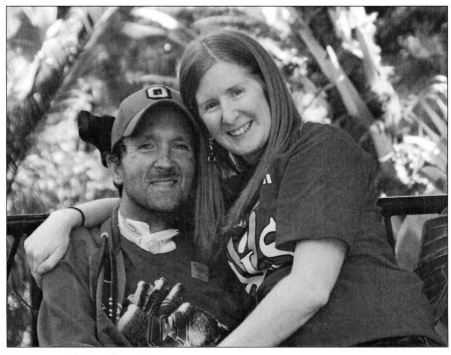

Matt June with his wife, Jackie.

As an avid baseball fan, Matt knew of the legend Lou Gehrig and the debilitating disease that bears his name. After his initial diagnosis, Matt was shocked and even depressed. Then came the doubt. "Could they be wrong?" With that motivation, Matt went to the Cleveland Clinic to get another opinion. It was confirmed; he had ALS. It took some time for the prognosis to sink in but then Matt had a revelation. He entered into the acceptance phase and determined to himself, "I can handle this."

Following this revelation, Matt went on a road trip with his oldest son, Mitch. It was July 2010 and Mitch was home on leave from the military. They drove from Ohio to Massachusetts, the state in which Mitch was born. From there, they drove down to Florida stopping to visit cities along the eastern seaboard until they landed in Tampa Bay, FL. The father and son stayed with Matt's best friend who arranged a big celebration party for his visitors. Matt and Mitch did not know anyone at the party but they felt at home. One particular woman, Jackie, caught Matt's eye with her slender build and her silky, strawberry-blonde hair. They hit it off and within six months, they were married.

Hungry to learn about the progression of ALS and to stay two steps ahead of its progress, Matt hunted the Internet to learn more. He became involved with an ALS online support community and would read frequent posts on the site. One post was attractive to Matt. It was written by a woman who described her Diaphragm Pacing System. ALS weakens the diaphragm of its victims causing insufficient oxygen into the lungs. This leads to a condition called chronic hypoventilation.

The **NeuRx DPS** (Diaphragm Pacing System) is a surgically implanted neurostimulation device that improves breathing for those with ALS and other conditions plagued with breathing problems. The system consists of four **PermaLoc** electrodes implanted into the diaphragm muscle with a fifth electrode implanted just under the skin.

The electrodes are grouped together into a socket called an electrode connector. The system is controlled through an external pulse generator (EPG), which connects to the socket using a removable cable.

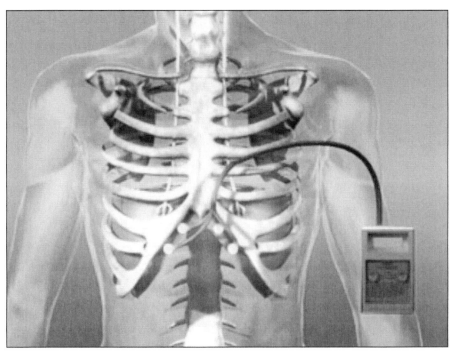

The NeuRx DPS consists of four electrodes implanted in the diaphragm to stimulate the muscle, a fifth electrode under the skin to complete the electrical circuit, a connector holder, a cable and an external battery-powered pulse generator. The pulse generator regulates movement of the diaphragm muscle, creating a vacuum-like effect in the chest cavity that draws air into the lungs. When this contraction eases, the air is expelled from the lungs. On average, this process is repeated 10 to 14 times per minute.

The EPG sends a signal to the electrodes then the electrodes stimulate the diaphragm muscle to contract. That contraction allows the lungs to fill or extract air. The operation is simple but the function is impactful.

ALS was starting to take a toll on Matt's body functions. While communicating in the on-line community about the DPS system, the mobility in his arms and legs started to decline. His symptoms led to him starting to use a power wheelchair. Reality of the progression of ALS was seeping into the newlyweds' lives. At that point, they knew they had to stay two steps ahead of the disease. The preservation of quality of life became a driving force for their future decisions.

Jackie and Matt reviewed their options for the DPS. They spoke with people who use the device to understand the process of getting one implanted. Medicare insurance would cover the device and the procedure. They concluded it would be a way for them to keep a quality of life for a longer time—the time they wanted together. And together they made the decision to have the system implanted into Matt's body.

Once they said "go," the process was fairly quick with minimal disruptions to their daily lives. On Sunday, Matt and Jackie drove to Cleveland to stay in a hotel near University Hospital at Case Western Reserve University. Monday, they were introduced to the surgeon, Dr. Raymond Onders, and the post-surgical team along with preliminary and preoperative testing. Tuesday was an open day. Wednesday morning Matt was admitted for the surgical procedure to take place late that morning with the remainder of the day for recovery. Thursday morning the medical team brought him the external components of the system, demonstrated the functions, and flipped the switch on the DPS. By Friday, they were driving back to Steubenville. With no anxiety, hesitation, or regret, Matt was now meeting his quest to preserve a quality of life. He and Jackie were reassured of this as they completed their journey back to Florida.

Even though getting the device was viewed as a preventative measure or more like a means to stave off the inevitable, Matt recognized that the device "became part of my body." When the symptoms of ALS started to progress, he viewed the DPS as a way of extending his time until he needed mechanical ventilation.

Much like a cardiac pacemaker, once the system is implanted there is minimal maintenance if it is used continuously. Approximately every three weeks, the EPG relays a warning for a weak battery, which indicates that it's time to change the size C lithium batteries. He has the comfort of knowing it is there when he needs it. Occasionally, he checks in with the medical team for the DPS. His oxygen saturation levels remained steady. As the disease progressed, some settings needed to be adjusted. His local Veterans Administration hospital had staff trained to help him with any needs or minor adjustments with the DPS.

Endeavoring to stay one step ahead of his disease is how Matt has approached his diagnosis. He has a level of acceptance of his diagnosis and the fate of the disease. It is a noble and courageous one. Matt's choices are based on his desire to be in control of his life rather than let the disease take over. When he was initially diagnosed he learned everything he could about the disease, its progress, and his options.

Matt knows that he will lose mobility, lose the ability to feed himself, and eventually lose his ability to breathe. He got the power wheelchair before it became a dire need. He will get the feeding tube before he can no longer feed himself. He had the DPS system implanted before he had symptoms that would require a mechanical ventilator. It's not that Matt was eager to accelerate the progression of his disease. Rather, he chose to exert some control on the journey he knew was forthcoming.

With that knowledge, he controls his quality of life and he has become a leader to help guide others with similar outcomes. He and Jackie are active in their ALS support group. It has helped him and he finds this as a way to give back to others. Every other month, they host a gathering of people living with ALS and their loved ones into their home. The time gives them an opportunity to reflect, interact, and converse with others in similar situations. It is a time to learn from each other the lessons that cannot be reviewed in a brochure or found through Google.

While using the DPS system, Matt has been able to remain as active as possible. He and his family engaged in a YOLO (You Only Live Once) summer tour. With his in-laws from England and three stepchildren, Jackie and Matt in his power wheelchair gathered into a minivan and drove over 3600 miles for a 17-day road tour. They went to places he always wanted to visit and shared them with his family. Starting in Florida, they visited destinations like Graceland in Tennessee, Mount Rushmore in South Dakota, Pikes Peak in Colorado, and the Grand Canyon in Arizona. It was an experience he always wanted to embrace. The joy, the adventure, and the sensations are what Matt uses to define his quality of life.

Bionic Pioneers

Chapter 9: Going Deep to Fight Parkinson's

The Story of Dr. Jonathan Lessin

Being dealt a card of a progressive neurological condition changes your perspective on life. Some neurological conditions can hit you like a brick wall while others creep into your life. This story is a combination of both aspects—the immediate impact and the slow progression of Parkinson's disease, a degenerative brain disorder. It is also the story of how one man changed his cards to gain a better quality of life.

It was five o'clock in the morning and Jonathan Lessin was driving to work to begin a busy day of surgeries. As a cardiac anesthesiologist, Dr. Lessin was living his dream. He had a great job, a wonderful wife, and two beautiful daughters. Although there was stress related to his job and long hours, he truly enjoyed his work.

During his early morning commute; Jonathan was waiting at an intersection for the red light to turn green. He was behind a large trunk stacked with ceramic tiles on its way to a construction site. Without warning a drunk driver traveling at 50 mph slammed into the back of Jonathan's car. He was sandwiched between the drunken driver who had fallen asleep at the wheel and the tile trunk. Jonathan was able to get out of his damaged vehicle but waited for two hours until the emergency crew arrived.

At age 33, the accident left him with a compression fracture in his spinal cord resulting in weakness on the right side of his body and a case of drop foot syndrome. He returned to the work that he loved and walked around using an ankle foot orthosis.

Five years later, the drop foot syndrome finally subsided and Jonathan was able to walk around without using the orthosis. But there were other strange symptoms starting to surface. He began to feel clumsy and noticed some difficulty with his handwriting and fine motor skills in his hands. The right side of his body began to feel stiffer and more rigid than his left side. Jonathan was walking slower and began bumping into things like revolving doors, a wall by a doorway, or even his car. Of course, any or all of these symptoms could have been residual effects from the car accident five years earlier. He was having issues, but he did not observe collective symptoms that would warrant a medical diagnosis.

One symptom finally surfaced that sparked Jonathan to seek medical assistance. He was pouring a Coke into a glass and observed his pinky finger quivering. That was it--a tremor. That tremor motivated Jonathan to seek the advice of a neurologist who was a friend of his wife's colleague.

Without any hesitation, the neurologist diagnosed Jonathan with Parkinson's disease. He was 38 years old. After receiving the news, there was a sense of relief. He was relieved to have a name associated with the strange symptoms he was experiencing. Ironically, for all the training Jonathan received in medical school, he learned very little about Parkinson's disease. During that training the focus was on tremors; no other symptoms were reviewed. Now that he had a diagnosis, he educated himself about the disease and ways to manage the symptoms.

The initial symptoms of Parkinson's disease can be very subtle and often do not surface until the symptoms reach an escalated level. People can have Parkinson's disease all their lives but they do not receive a diagnosis until a sufficient number of neurons in the brain begin to be impacted. At that point, the outward symptoms begin to surface. For Jonathan, his diagnosis pulled together all the symptoms he was experiencing.

Regardless of his diagnosis, he still did not believe it. He still could not come to terms that he had the disease. Jonathan was in denial.

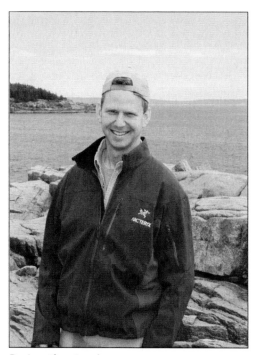

Dr. Jonathan Lessin

As was customary, Jonathan sought a second opinion and he was diagnosed with the same condition, Parkinson's disease. Still not fully accepting the fact that he had the disease, Jonathan went through the actions to begin treatment. There are several different types of medications for Parkinson's disease. As Jonathan began taking them, his symptoms were not improving. He remained in denial, believing that if the medications were not working then he must not have the disease. But eventually, one of the medications started to treat his symptoms. One pill worked. With that one pill improving Jonathan's symptoms, he could no longer be in denial. He had Parkinson's disease.

Accepting his diagnosis, Jonathan began to educate himself about the disease and inventory his options. Being an anesthesiologist helped with his quest. One of his options for the treatment of Parkinson's disease is a medical device called a deep brain stimulation (DBS) system. Several times in the past, Jonathan had been the anesthesiologist during surgeries to implant DBS devices. He was familiar with the surgical implantation process and how the device relieved tremors but he was not familiar with how it could impact the patients who were receiving them. Even with this knowledge, Jonathan accepted the medical advice and began the typical pharmaceutical regime of taking a myriad of medications

These medications work in three different stages: UNDER, ON, or OVER. The goal is to be in the ON stage for as long as possible. This is when the chemical balance is close enough to normal that the symptoms subside. Prior to this stage, he is in the UNDER stage while waiting for the medication to take effect.

Before the drugs took effect, Jonathan felt very stiff and rigid. He also had the feeling of carrying massive weight on his arms and legs. As the medications began to take effect, he then progressed to the ON stage. In this state, Jonathan was able move around as he did before and felt a sense of relief, as if weight was lifted off his arms and legs. The ON stage clicked for Jonathan like a light switch going from OFF to ON.

After the ON stage, he progresses to the OVER stage. This is when the medication is working but too much. Jonathan would have extraordinary movements and wait for the medication to slowly wear down to try to reach the ON stage again. The roller coaster between the three stages is a daily routine and a delicate chemical balance to control the symptoms of the disease. The result is a very small amount of time during the day when Jonathan was in the ON stage. At that point, he began to exhaust his options for the pharmaceutical regime.

During this progression, Jonathan had seen news stories on NBC's Dateline and CBS 60 minutes highlighting the DBS technology commonly used to treat symptoms of Parkinson's disease such as tremors, rigidity, stiffness, and slowed movements. DBS is a surgically implanted system consisting of three components: the electrode lead, an extension, and a neurostimulator. The lead is inserted through a small opening in the skull and placed in a precise target in the brain, which may be the subthalamic nucleus or the globus pallidus interna. The surgeons typically use microelectrode recordings to determine the optimal placement of the electrode lead. The lead is connected to the extension, which is an insulated wire tunneled under the skin of the head, neck, and shoulder. The extension connects to the neurostimulator, which is typically implanted under the skin in the collarbone area. The neurostimulator is a battery powered medical device similar to a heart pacemaker. Once the system is implanted and operational, the neurostimulator delivers electrical signals through the extension to the lead electrode. These signals or pulses to the targeted area in the brain interfere with or block the abnormal nerve activity that cause tremors and other symptoms related to Parkinson's disease.

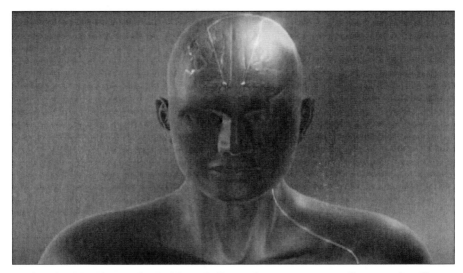

Medtronic's DBS Therapy for Parkinson's disease incorporates a small, pacemaker-like device that sends electronic signals to an area in the brain that controls movement. These signals block some of the brain messages that cause annoying and disabling motor symptoms. The device is placed under the skin in the chest. Very thin wires connect the device to the brain to enable the signals to reach the source of the symptoms. (Image courtesy of Medtronic Inc.)

As Jonathan began to do his research about DBS, he watched video after video on the Internet of DBS success stories. Not all of the videos were success stories. Jonathan watched one video about a man for whom DBS was not successful and he had the device removed.

In his research, Jonathan educated himself about the system, how it works, the surgical procedure, the complication rates and he spoke with other doctors regarding DBS technology. He went to medical centers like the Cleveland Clinic and Georgetown to gather more information. As he learned more, Jonathan began to wonder why his neurologist did not provide DBS as an option for him earlier. Jonathan decided to ask. He approached his neurologist with an inquiry as to whether he would be a candidate for the technology. Once Jonathan asked, his neurologist agreed that he would be good candidate.

From Jonathan's point of view, his neurologist did not mention the option since most people are afraid of brain surgery and the potential risks associated with it. The thought of opening up your skull to implant a medical device can be disconcerting. As a result, people tend to wait until they are desperate and out of other options before receiving a DBS system. Jonathan was no different.

By the time he scheduled the surgery, he could no longer function using medications. He had lost 50 pounds mainly due to his diet restrictions. For Jonathan, he had to avoid protein in his diet since protein would block the dopamine and his body would go stiff. He had to avoid foods like soy sauce, turkey, and peanut butter. He began losing weight rapidly due to his restricted diet of mainly vegetables and crackers. The turning point for Jonathan was when his wife, Cheryl, bought a juicer and was pureeing celery for him to take. At that point, he knew something had to change.

Jonathan also tried to continue to work but at times the symptoms were so bad he could not perform his job, even with accommodation from his employer. Instead, he was forced to take vacation time while he attempted to better manage the debilitating symptoms of Parkinson's disease. As he became more resistant to the medications, his symptoms began to impact every aspect of his life. He was no longer able to work much less perform basic activities of daily living.

For Jonathan, DBS was an option he couldn't deny. "Once I get my wires, I'll be able to function, he told himself."

Getting the system implanted requires several steps. The first step is to identify the placement of the electrode lead. Jonathan went through the pre-operative testing using magnetic resonance imaging (MRI) to locate the exact target within the brain where the neural signals generate the symptoms of Parkinson's disease. In the operating room, Jonathan's head was placed into a frame while the lead electrode and the extension wire were surgically placed into the brain. Once the implantation surgery was complete, Jonathan had a post-operative computed tomography (CT) scan to confirm the placement of the lead then waited three weeks for his body to heal. The next step was to surgically implant the battery-powered neurostimulator. The final step was activating the system and customizing the program for Jonathan's specific anatomy.

The day that the system was activated was a vivid day for Jonathan. His appointment was for one o'clock in the afternoon. That morning, he could not take any of his medications and his body reacted to the lack of medications. His symptoms were severe and Jonathan's body became stiffer and stiffer. At one point, he could hardly move. He went to the hospital early with the escort of his parents. His doctor came into the waiting room and said, "Come with me." Somehow, Jonathan was able to get up from the waiting room chair and follow the doctor. It was time to activate the system; one side at a time. His doctor activated one side and immediately the stiffness in Jonathan's muscles melted away. Excited, he began running around the clinic, "This is amazing!" His doctor had to gather Jonathan back to the examining room to activate the second side.

Once the system is activated, the settings are adjusted

for optimum performance to Jonathan's brain. Since the brain is a fluid environment and there is scar tissue from the surgery the system programming may need to be adjusted several times. This was the case for Jonathan.

Each month after the surgery, Jonathan would visit his neurologist for a system adjustment, which would include changing a parameter such as pulse width or current. On the ninth month, it clicked. His neurologist made an adjustment and the system began to work perfectly. Jonathan could feel it instantly and he knew they now had the perfect setting for his specific needs. He was also given a small remote so he could make minor adjustments to the program to meet his daily needs.

Jonathan was familiar and comfortable with the surgical procedure, particularly due to his medical background. Regardless, he still had concerns about potential surgical risks such as bleeding, infection, or cognitive side effects.

His bigger decision was not whether to get the DBS system but where to have the surgery. What was more dramatic for him was how the system felt. "The system goes from OFF to ON," he explained. After the system has been programmed to meet Jonathan's customized needs, it does all the work for him. He affectionately calls it "gumption." It is the feeling that the system is working and he has the freedom to move when he wants to and a platform to support his daily activities.

He believes that his core muscles have gotten stronger and he knows that he can move when he wants rather than waiting for the medication to create the proper balance. With DBS, he feels in control rather than the medications controlling him. Prior to surgery, Jonathan was taking medications every two hours; now, he only takes them three times per day. The system is rechargeable. Since

Jonathan uses his system at a high level, he recharges his batteries about three times per week.

Once he received his DBS, he only wished he received it sooner. The surgery day was a significant day in Jonathan's life. After his wedding day and the birth of his children, getting the DBS was "the best day of my life." The DBS system gives him a new freedom of movement that was strangled by Parkinson's disease. With his improved movement, he is able to exercise and has become healthier, regaining the weight he lost earlier. He can now eat protein and enjoys his beloved ice cream, including a banana split. Sleep deprivation is a common occurrence for people living with Parkinson's disease. With the DBS, Jonathan can sleep more comfortably and throughout the night. There are subtle changes as well. His wife noticed the return of his facial expressions.

More dramatic is Jonathan's return to an active lifestyle. Although he retired from his medical practice, he now is an enthusiastic indoor rock climber, scaling walls three times per week. An avid skier, Jonathan was able to return to the slopes—even the more challenging mogul runs. The past winter, he went to the Breckenridge Winter Sports Center in Colorado and joined a program specifically for people living with Parkinson's disease. There, he had some of the best skiing in his life, even prior to being diagnosed. He can't specifically say his performance was due to the DBS system, but he knows that he would not be able to step foot on the ski slope without the system.

While conducting his research before being implanted with the DBS system, Jonathan came across some of the earlier medical research studies regarding implantation of DBS within the early stages of Parkinson's disease. The medical research supports using the device as an early intervention rather than a final option. When he was diagnosed Jonathan was in the first stage of Parkinson's disease. Nearly 10 years later, he is now in the second stage. He believes that he could easily be in the third or fourth and final stages of Parkinson's disease if he did not have the DBS system.

Jonathan inspires others to be informed about Parkinson's disease, DBS, and other options for treating the symptoms of the disease. He encourages others to visit the National Parkinson's Disease website and find the National Parkinson's Disease Foundation Center of Excellence medical centers. These specialty centers can provide guidance about what to expect with Parkinson's disease and explain DBS along with the risks and benefits.

Jonathan has discovered that exercise helps to relieve his symptoms. With his DBS system, he learned how to adjust his system using the small remote. With this he gets better performance by adjusting to his daily needs. Jonathan also encourages others living with Parkinson's disease not to wait until they are desperate to begin looking for alternative solutions to pharmaceutical treatments. The earlier in the diagnosis for interventions like DBS, the better one will be in the long run.

Jonathan turned his clumsiness into inspiration. "When you are diagnosed with Parkinson's disease, what was once known as clumsy is now inspirational," he said.

Bionic Pioneers

Chapter 10: Unlocking the Brain

The Story of Cathy Hutchinson

Imagine suddenly living inside the body of a mannequin. All of your movements are frozen, but your senses remain active. You can see, smell, hear, and feel but you can't respond to any of them, neither by movement, expression, nor speech. Your mind is functioning perfectly. You are observing the outside world but not able to interact with it or anyone.

This is just one way to describe locked-in syndrome (LIS). It's a "rare" condition. The condition may be caused from a variety of sources such as traumatic brain injury, disease, or more commonly, stroke. The options are scarce for people living in a locked-in body. Meet one woman who is trail-blazing the way to give those with LIS an outlet to the world.

Cathy Hutchinson was a 43-year-old single parent living in Massachusetts with her two teenage children, Brian and Holly. Due to her heavy work schedule and involvement with her children, Cathy seldom had time for hobbies outside of her home. The one exception was her garden. It was a place where she enjoyed getting her hands dirty, feeling the soil between her fingers, and sampling the fruits (and vegetables) of her labor. Her friends would declare that she was "a slave to her garden," since any spare moment would lead her back to it. Tending to her garden was a way for her to relax and find solitude in an, otherwise hectic lifestyle.

On a spring afternoon, Cathy and her son, Brian, were preparing the soil for some new plants and seeds. Brian was doing the heavy lifting while Cathy was grooming the soil for fresh vegetable plants. Wanting some respite from the heavy lifting, Brian asked if they could take a break. He wanted to go inside the house to view the basketball game and get an update on the score. Cathy conceded, brushed off the excess dirt and joined Brian in the house.

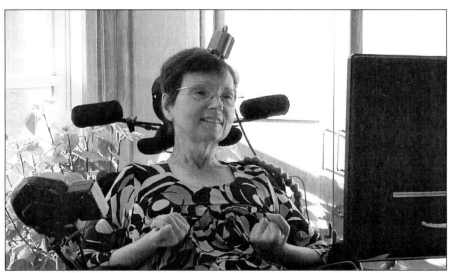

Cathy Hutchinson

Once inside, Cathy suddenly felt nauseous. She told Brian that she was going upstairs to her bedroom. After climbing the stairway, Cathy's right foot began to shake violently, her body collapsed and she fainted to the floor. Brian heard the sound and ran up the steps. Finding his mother on the floor, Brian made a makeshift bed for her to lay on until he could get professional help.

Cathy was in and out of consciousness, but while lying on the floor staring at the ceiling, she knew she had had a stroke. She did not know why or how she knew. The symptoms she was experiencing were related to a stroke and she simply knew. What she did not know was the depth of the danger it presented.

Cathy could hear Brian calling her sister, Dottie, and then calling for an ambulance. Cathy's daughter, Holly, was working at the shopping mall and would be home soon. Cathy did not want her to come home to an ambulance outside her home. Fortunately, the ambulance arrived before Holly did. Cathy did not want to go into the ambulance, but Dottie convinced her to proceed. Once again, Cathy began to feel weak and dizzy. With assistance from the EMT crew, Cathy went into the ambulance and was reluctantly transported to the local hospital. That was the last time she could walk or talk.

Admitted to the hospital immediately, the doctors confirmed what Cathy already knew. She had had a stroke, a brain stem stroke. The brain stem is located above the spinal cord and it controls many involuntary functions such as breathing and blood pressure. Nerves controlling eye movement, talking, swallowing, and muscle movement, are within or routed through the brain stem. A brain stem stroke occurs when the blood supply is interrupted, nerve cells are damaged, and the person is left with a life-threatening situation.

For Cathy, her body needed to be stabilized but she was left with locked-in syndrome. Later, she was moved to a rehabilitation hospital in Braintree, MA. Through their patient training program, Cathy began to learn how to communicate using only eye movements and blinks. They also offered patient education classes to help her understand the causes and effects of stroke. This made Cathy even more curious.

How could this be medically possible? Cathy was not a chronic smoker. She smoked when she was a teenager, 30 years earlier, but not now. She had low blood pressure and cholesterol. There was no family history of a stroke or stroke-type symptoms. Hereditary seems to be the only culprit but Cathy refused to accept it. With some additional research, she found that a stroke can be caused by heart disease.

Along with learning how to adapt to being locked inside a completely paralyzed body, Cathy would experience extreme and uncontrollable emotions. For instance, she would begin to laugh inappropriately and hysterically for no reason. This condition of uncontrollable emotions became very annoying to her but also intrigued her curiosity. She initially suspected that was due to depression but later discovered that as a result of the stroke, she developed a condition called Pseudobulbar affect (PBA). According to the National Stroke Association, PBA is a medical condition in which people have sudden and uncontrollable episodes of crying or laughing that can occur at any time, even within inappropriate social situations.

The culmination of being locked-in a paralyzed body, unable to communicate with the outside world, and having uncontrollable emotions led Cathy to no longer live independently. From all of this, the most devastating experience for her was the role reversal. As a divorced parent, Cathy was always taking care of her children, but now the roles were reversed. Her sisters volunteered to help by opening their homes to Brian and Holly and assisting

Cathy with her insurance and finances. They gave Cathy one job, recovery.

Directly after her stroke, Cathy could communicate with her eyes only. Once she was transferred to a rehabilitation hospital, her physical therapist began working with her to see what they could recover. With much patience and an abundance of encouragement, Cathy left the hospital for an assisted living facility. She had the ability to hold her head up and respond by shaking her head. She also used a head tracker to operate a computer, allowing her to communicate with staff and surf the web. Her method of communication was via a manual board with eye tracking, but it was laborious. Each word needed to be spelled out. Unless she was with someone who knew how to use the board, she could not communicate at all.

Cathy's experience as a stroke survivor was frustrating. Frustrating by not being able to say what she wanted to say, to move when she wanted to move, and to care for those people and things that she loved. All of her freedom was lost. She slipped into depression for short periods but she was frustrated at the situation she found herself. All of her experiences were not just frustrating; some were humorous at times. Some people who do not know Cathy or have not worked with her tend to assume that since she is paralyzed and nonverbal then she is not cognitively functional or aware of her surroundings.

Moving to a new hospital was concerning for Cathy since none of the staff knew her with the exception of the nurse supervisor. Upon Cathy's arrival, she heard a familiar voice, "Cathy, do you remember me?" shouted the nurse in excitement. She gave Cathy a warm greeting and assured her that she would inform the staff about her needs, abilities, and preferences with her admission to the hospital.

Meanwhile, Cathy was getting settled into her new room when a nurse's aide came into her room with breakfast. The aide did not greet Cathy. In fact, she did not talk to her at all. She did not ask Cathy how she preferred her coffee or whether she wanted her banana separately or in her cereal. Instead, the aide picked up the banana off Cathy's breakfast tray. She then proceeded to peel back the skin, take a bite of the banana and place it back onto the tray. Cathy watched in astonishment.

The aide then began to feed Cathy some eggs when the nurse supervisor came into the room and introduced Cathy to the aide. The supervisor explained that she had taken care of Cathy when she first had her stroke several years earlier. She then said, "This is Cathy. Although she cannot move or speak, she is well aware of her surroundings. She is very observant and does not miss a trick." Cathy then looked at the aide and smiled. With a blushing face of a brilliant red, the aide quickly looked to the floor. But Cathy was not angry. Instead, she was laughing inside. True laughter is essential for a healthy recovery. She finds humor in every challenge or situation. That is how she survives.

Aside from her survival mechanisms, the inability to talk to people is more frustrating than not being able to move. Knowing this led Paula, Cathy's best friend, on a quest to find an alternative communication tool. As a hospital quality management coordinator, Paula learned about a neural prosthesis research project specifically for people with conditions similar to Cathy. Her best friend found the intake doctor's name and advocated for Cathy. Paula persisted until she had the right connections. Her persistence would lead Cathy on a five-year journey filled with excitement and knowledge. Her journey would be with the BrainGate research team.

BrainGate is a clinical and technology research effort with the ultimate goal of helping people with spinal cord injury, stroke, muscular dystrophy, ALS, limb loss, or other injuries or illnesses to restore their mobility, communication, and independence. The BrainGate investigational technology is being developed to detect brain signals and to allow people with paralysis to use those signals or thoughts to control assistive devices. The system is based on neuroscience, engineering and computer science research conducted by a multidisciplinary research team at Massachusetts General Hospital, Brown University, Providence Veterans Administration Medical Center, and other institutions. For Cathy and others with locked-in syndrome, the ability to easily communicate is a high priority.

The BrainGate system has three main components: the sensor, decoder, and external device. The sensor is a 4x4 millimeter 100-element electrode array that is surgically implanted into the motor cortex of the brain. The decoder component consists of a set of computers with software that converts brain signals into useful commands. The third component, the external device, can be any number of assistive devices are capable of accepting electronic signals and using those signals to perform a useful function. These include a communication device, electric wheelchair, or a robotic limb.

The three components are coordinated together to give a natural interaction with the outside world. The sensor records neural action potentials from the brain and sends the signals to the decoder. The decoder translates the brain signals into actionable commands. Those commands are sent to the external device producing the desired output.

Cathy learned about the BrainGate technology from Paula and immediately wanted to participate. Paula made the initial call to discuss general information about the clinical trial. That was followed by a two-minute telephone questionnaire to see if Cathy met the inclusion and exclusion criteria and could be a potential candidate. There was some hesitation from the research team regarding Cathy's current condition and her ability to give feedback as a research participant. But Paula persisted that Cathy was the ideal candidate for this research. Again her persuasion convinced the team to consider Cathy and follow up with a third interview conducted in-person with members of the research team to further discuss the expectations of the study and to address any questions. Passing the first three litmus tests, Cathy enrolled and advanced to the final medical screening tests and an MRI of her brain.

Eager to become an active participant in a clinical trial, Cathy was ready for something new. She was completely ignorant of the technology but excited to learn about it as a potential new window to the world; a new communication interface to ease the laborious exercise of asking for her coffee using a manual board. She was now optimistic about what the future may hold for her.

Clinical trials with new technology typically take time, effort, and support on the part of the participant. For Cathy, time was not a concern since she now had plenty of it. The effort that she would put into the trial gave her new motivation in life. The financial commitment was a concern but it was calmed as she was reassured that there would be no monetary outlay on her part. Reviewing the same information that Cathy had, her son, Brian, voiced two concerns about the technology. First, would his mom have brain damage from the implant? Second, would this impact her memory? Those concerns were addressed as he became aware of the risks and the safety testing of the technology, particularly those that are implanted into the human body. With that reassurance, her family fully supported her participation. She now had a new window opened from her imprisonment for several years.

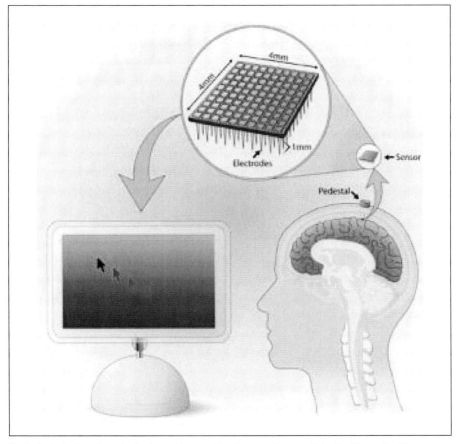

BrainGate technology is designed to read brain signals associated with controlling movement, which a computer could translate into instructions for moving a computer cursor or controlling a variety of assistive devices. The BrainGate neural interface system consists of a sensor to monitor brain signals and computer software and hardware that turns these signals into digital commands for external devices. The sensor is a baby aspirin-sized square of silicon containing 100 hair-thin electrodes, which can record the activity of small groups of brain cells. It is implanted into the motor cortex, a part of the brain that directs movement. (Image courtesy of Brown Institute for Brain Science)

Cathy's surgery date finally arrived. Filled with excitement, she awaited the team to take her to the operating room for the implanting of the microelectrode array into her brain. Sedated for the experience, the neurosurgeons carefully placed the device on Cathy's motor cortex, tested the electrode for proper placement, and verified that it was capturing the needed signals. Her incisions were sutured and they sent Cathy off to the recovery room. By the next day, Cathy was up in her electric wheelchair and driving it around the hospital, leaving the staff astonished by her rapid recovery.

With the surgical and recovery phase completed, it was now time to allow Cathy to use the system in real-time. The laboratory was mobile and came to Cathy. The research team transported the computers humming and pre-programmed but missing one critical piece. Cathy was holding the key component to make the system flow. The research team connected a wire from the computer to the port on her head, essentially linking the brain implant to the computer. They gave her some instructions for the first exercise to test the system using her thoughts to move a cursor on the computer screen. Without further explanation, Cathy knew what to do instantly; the implant would make the connection from her intentions to actionable movement on the screen in front of her. She wanted to move the cursor left. She would think about her fisted hand moving left and in coordinated fashion, the cursor would move left. The delay from her thought to the cursor moving was a matter of just milliseconds.

The process felt natural. The first time she saw the cursor move across the screen, she could not believe her eyes. But she wanted more. She kept moving the cursor across the screen. She was elated. One of the engineers asked

Cathy if she was in control. With her approval, they then gave her an active screen keyboard. He asked her, "What month is it?" With ease, Cathy chose her letters to spell "J-U-L-Y" on the screen. At that point she knew she was in control. It was the most jaw-dropping experience of her life.

Her natural progression sparked the research team to elevate the challenges they presented to Cathy. Since she had mastered the movement of a cursor and the on-screen keyboard, the team gave her the challenge of managing environmental controls, like lighting, music, or drapery. This was no challenge for her. For each new challenge, Cathy would return to her room satisfied that she made the right decision of being a clinical trial participant.

The research team then upped the ante. That day, Cathy approached the mobile laboratory with great enthusiasm as she was excited to move the technology forward to a more complex task. For this exercise, the assistive device was an electric wheelchair. The team would ask Cathy to control this empty wheelchair simply by thought. They turned the reins over to her and she gave a signal to move the wheelchair forward and then in reverse. The task went exactly as planned. Cathy had complete control of moving the wheelchair around an open area.

Ready to take the next challenge, the research team asked Cathy to drive the wheelchair toward one of the investigators and then through a doorway. She proceeded but with a few more hiccups. As the wheelchair approached the investigator, Cathy felt like she lost control and panicked. The wheelchair nearly ran over the investigator's foot. Feeling horrified and disappointed, Cathy looked up at the faces of the research team. They were laughing. Cathy could only laugh along with them. Once again, humor was her best coping mechanism.

This one incident did not stop the progress. Her next challenge would launch Cathy into the limelight. With the same sensor and decoder, the research team added a more complex assistive device, a multi-directional robotic hand and arm. To begin using this new tool, a member of the research team moved the arm while Cathy thought of that movement. She was training to think about moving her own arm while the decoder was adapting to understand her thought patterns. These adaptations would convert to algorithms to get the desired output to the robotic arm. Once Cathy and the system were working in unison, she began to use the robotic arm and hand on her own. "I was in control of my right arm and hand. It felt normal again, natural and comfortable," Cathy recalled.

As the research team was improving the system response, movements, and communication interfaces. Cathy was visiting the lab to test the latest developments of the full system. Gradually, the robotic arm was able to perform functional tasks for Cathy. She adores her morning coffee, more specifically a cinnamon latte. Typically, a caregiver must position the cup in a holder by Cathy's mouth while she sips from a straw. On this day, Cathy manipulated the robotic arm to pick up her coffee, bring it to her and hold it while she drank her cinnamon latte. For the first time in 15 years, Cathy was drinking her coffee independently. For her, it was the most delicious cinnamon latte she had ever tasted. For the research team, they witnessed the most beautiful smile they had ever seen. The video of Cathy performing this somewhat simple task went viral around the world.

Days passed and years slipped by. Cathy spent five years working with the BrainGate technology. At the end of the trial, the implanted micro-array was removed from

Cathy's body. She had entered the clinical trial with the understanding that there was an endpoint. Her means of communication, environmental control, and use of assistive devices via thought had now ceased. But the research team did not allow her to return to the laborious communication board, they provided her with a more robust communication tool. Using eye gaze technology and a new radial electronic keyboard, this mobile tool allows Cathy to communicate quickly and efficiently. After using the technology for several months, Cathy is convinced it will replace the QWERTY keyboard. It was offered to her by the Speak Your Mind Foundation, speakyourmindfoundation.org. All of this excites Cathy to continue participating in clinical trials. If she was asked to participate again, she would not hesitate to take part in the research process again.

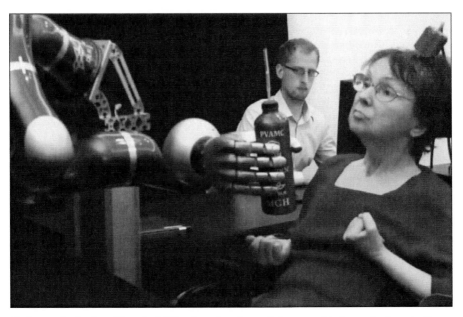

Cathy made the headlines in 2012 when she showed she was able to control a robotic arm using the BrainGate system. (Photo courtesy of The BrainGate Collaboration)

Cathy shares:

"I can't take credit for progress I have made in my recovery. I have been blessed with doctors, therapists, and caregivers. My sisters, Geri and Dottie, have supported me since the beginning. I will always be grateful to them and love them both dearly. If not for the research trial and assistive technology, I could not have made the recovery. It is still an on-going process. This research and the assistive devices have made my life a lot less frustrating. I am able to get through the daily challenges."

During her five-year journey in the BrainGate study, Cathy saw equipment upgrades, software renditions, and adaptive equipment experiments. Along the way, she learned about herself, discovered her slow recovery, and experienced cutting edge technology converting thought into functional actions--including sipping the most delicious cinnamon latte. Researchers are on the threshold of a new generation of technology. Scientists need more volunteers to be part of the revolution. It is up to these brave pioneers to make it happen.

Chapter 11: A Stroke of Good Luck

The Story of Linda Gordon

The human brain is a frontier of discovery. In recent years, conventional scientific beliefs about the brain have been challenged by the notion of neural plasticity. Plasticity is defined as the natural capability of the brain to "rewire" itself, to form new neural connections, and to reassign the function of existing neurons within the brain.

The details of this process are still the subject of scientific exploration. In the meantime, how can this phenomenon be used to impact people today? How can we capitalize on the presence of plasticity to improve recovery, eradicate disorders, or accelerate the rehabilitation process? This story is about a woman who is using a device to improve her condition even though the device was originally designed for a very different application.

Linda faced a typical day of work as a customer adviser on January 11, 2012. Her morning routine was ordinary, as was her morning commute. Nothing seemed unusual to her for most of the morning. But as the day progressed, Linda started to notice some abnormalities in her ability to perform her job. Suddenly, she had difficulty writing. Even so, she did not have grave concerns. It could have been a cramp or other circumstance related to getting older. As a woman in her mid-50's, she knew there are occasional aches and pains that can occur. This must have been one of those instances.

It was not until a colleague observed that Linda had slurred speech and a staggering gait that a more serious condition become even remotely possible. Putting the symptoms together—difficulty writing, slurred speech, and imbalance while walking—it was more than a simple ache or pain. At that point, Linda's friend and colleague took her straight to the hospital.

By the time they arrived at the hospital and through the admission process, Linda felt just fine, but the physicians did not concur. Her condition became progressively worse. Linda was admitted as an in-patient to the hospital for additional testing. Later consulted by her treating physician, Linda was told that she had not one but a series of three strokes. As a result, she had paralysis on one side of her body, the right side. This condition is known as hemiparesis and is a common result of traumatic stroke. Her rehabilitation from the incident would be long and the prospects were unknown. That one hospital stay stretched to four weeks.

In some sense, hospitals can be comforting, particularly when living with a new disability. They are comforting because as you learn how to live with an acquired disability such as paralysis, the space is known. You know how wide the doorway may be or the accessibility of the bathroom. Even if you don't, the medical staff is available to help when you need it.

Going home is another scenario. A place that you once knew and cherished becomes an obstacle you may not be expecting. The fact is that the home has not changed, but you have. Learning to live in your own home in different circumstances can prove to be difficult.

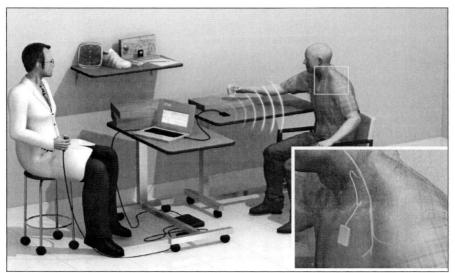

MicroTransponder's Vivistim System has been developed to treat stroke patients that experience an upper-limb deficit following their stroke. The system includes an implanted vagus nerve stimulation (VNS) system, a wireless transmitter, and targeted therapy sessions. Each therapy session involves a series of tasks and each task is repeated several times. MicroTransponder believes that short bursts of VNS paired with rehabilitation movements promotes plasticity in the brain and will improve arm weakness after stroke. (Image courtesy of MicroTransponder Inc.)

This was the case for Linda. The transition from hospital room to her home was strenuous. Her husband of 35 years, Alistair, was there to help her. The common place of her home was now an obstacle. The home that she knew so well was now different. Her home where she raised her two children and nurtured her four grandchildren was now difficult to navigate.

Linda came to realize that simple tasks she once took for granted were now impossible or extremely difficult to perform. Stairs were an overwhelming obstruction, particularly because all the bedrooms and bathrooms were on the second floor. The time to climb those stairs increased exponentially from what she could do in just a matter of seconds a few months prior. Climbing those stairs, Linda became acutely aware that there are common tasks that she could no longer do in her post-stroke, hemiparetic body.

Life was a challenge with the use of only one side of her body. As a right-handed person, Linda had to learn how to do everything with only her left hand. Trying to get dressed with only one hand became a laborious task. At first thought, it might be easy but in practice it is quite difficult. Try to zip a jacket or tie a shoe. She attempted to write with her left hand with no success. It was a frustrating situation under which she was powerless. Unable to write and with half her body paralyzed, Linda stopped working. This was just one more piece of her life that had been disrupted by the stroke.

With her standard physiotherapy completed and struggling with daily tasks at home, Linda had run out of options to try to improve until she received a telephone call from her daughter. Her daughter had read an advertisement in the newspaper about a new therapy for stroke survivors and they were looking to recruit patients. After reading the advertisement, her daughter encouraged Linda to at least inquire to see if she might be a candidate. Linda was hesitant and later discussed it with her husband, Alistair. "Go ahead, call, and inquire. What do you have to lose?" he advised.

The advertisement was recruiting stroke survivors to participate in a clinical trial. The trial would be using proven technology but in a very different way. Vagus nerve stimulation is used and has been proven safe for conditions such as epilepsy and depression. The device is implanted into the body and consists of a small electrode wrapped around the vagus nerve on the left side of the neck and also a small matchbook-size receiver implanted in the upper chest area. Through the use of a wireless remote, the implanted receiver sends signals to the electrode. The electrode stimulates the vagus nerve, which sends signals to the brain. For this trial, participants would receive the implanted vagus nerve stimulation system coupled with physiotherapy. The focus of the therapy is on hand and arm function for stroke survivors who have upper extremity paralysis or impairment. The treatment focuses on capitalizing on the plasticity of the brain.

Linda's inquiry led her to consider participating in the trial. Although there are risks with any surgical procedure, it seemed to be safe. Vagus nerve stimulators are implanted in thousands of people around the world. The prospect of having one more option to help improve her condition was uplifting. She had drop shoulder—paralysis from her shoulder down to her fingertips with no sensation or movement. This trial offered some hope for her. If she did nothing, then she would always wonder if the technology could have helped her. "Nothing lost, nothing gained." With that thought, Linda stepped forward and decided to become a participant in the clinical trial.

She again called the telephone number from the newspaper advertisement and made an appointment for a thorough evaluation. Upon her arrival at the medical center, she went through the intake paperwork and a plethora of tests to see if she met the criteria and qualified to be a participant. During that visit, the staff explained the technology in detail as well as the surgical procedure. She and Alistair were introduced to the research team, the treatment protocol, and the expectation for her commitment to the therapy. The information was thorough, the prospects were exciting, and the experience a bit overwhelming. But in the end, Linda was ready to join the trial.

A few weeks passed after her whirlwind visit to the medical center when she received the call. Linda was accepted into the trial and she would step into an experimental treatment option for her upper extremity paralysis. Three weeks after her acceptance, Linda returned to the medical center. This return was for the surgical procedure to implant the vagus nerve stimulation system. The procedure left her with a small incision on her neck and one on her upper chest between her collarbone and breast. By the next day, she was released to go home for the healing process.

That process took one month, after which she returned to visit the doctor for a follow-up from the procedure. He confirmed that everything had healed properly and she may proceed to the next stage of the protocol. Linda began physiotherapy for one hour three times per week. During each session, the clinical team would activate the stimulation system using a computer. This would send electrical impulses to the vagus nerve while she performed exercises with her impaired right arm and hand.

When they first turned the system on, Linda could feel the stimulation. It was an odd feeling but not painful or uncomfortable. Many of the exercises were repetitive tasks such as opening and closing her hand but some consisted of stretching her right arm. Once the session was complete, the stimulator would remain dormant. Access to the facility was relatively convenient since it was only 25 minutes from her home. Once the physiotherapy sessions were completed, Linda continued with her ongoing exercise program to perform at home without the stimulation.

The theory behind this treatment method is that the vagus nerve stimulation will lead to the release neurotransmitters to the brain. The stimulation, coupled with targeted, repetitive exercises, will result in further functional gains than just exercise alone.

The treatment method is still being proven by research. But for Linda, the results are real. Six months after completing the stimulation treatments and performing her exercises at home, Linda can now move her right arm, hand, and fingers. The movement is not as it was prior to her strokes but that movement allows her to have more function at home. Linda can now pick things up using her right hand. That movement translates to meaningful activities like feeding herself. Dressing is no longer as laborious with the use of both her hands. Gaining the use of her right hand allows Linda to be more independent even in her own home.

Now that two years have passed since the day of her multiple strokes, Linda reflects and has seen marked improvements. Before she participated in this research trial, her right arm was in a sling and completely paralyzed. Now, she has nearly full range of motion in her arm. She admittedly still needs some improvement in her elbow and fine finger movements, but functional improvements are impactful.

Although the trial is ongoing and following her progress over the long term, Linda's treatment sessions are complete. She still wonders whether it was the stimulation or simply the exercises that helped her gain the improvements in her right arm and hand. Regardless, Linda is happy that she received the call from her daughter and happy she became a participant. She is glad that she looked into this research trial particularly when there were no other options.

Chapter 12: Future Outlook

In the previous chapters, we've seen some excellent examples of how bionic pioneers have helped blaze the trail for neurotechnology therapies. In this final chapter, we'll look ahead at what may lie in store for neurotechnology users in the years ahead. We'll also examine some of the issues confronting neurotechnology users, researchers, clinicians, and the industry, as they forge ahead with new therapies and treatments to improve the quality of our lives.

Last Resort Syndrome

No matter how promising neurotechnology therapies appear to be, the field is often confronted with a serious handicap: the perception that neurotech therapies should only be an option after every other available therapy has been tried without success. Indeed, when a new neurotech therapy is approved by the FDA, it is often labeled as only for individuals who have failed to respond to conventional therapy, usually pharmaceuticals. These treatment-resistant, or "refractory" patients are often the hardest to treat and the ones who need therapy the most.

An interesting example of this attitude among users and clinicians comes to us from the field of cochlear implants, where an implanted neurostimulation device has restored hearing to hundreds of thousands of deaf people. When radio talk show host Rush Limbaugh announced to the world that he had lost his hearing in 2002, he said that before he could even be considered a candidate for a cochlear implant, he went through months of "traditional" therapy with drugs aimed at treating or reversing his auto immune inner ear disease.

"I'm popping pills [and] I'm shooting up stuff," he said on the air before receiving his implant. "I've never done stuff like this before. If this stuff doesn't work, then there is one other option that is relatively new, but it's not something that has been done enough to where a pattern has been established to say that it's acceptable. There's always the last resort—the cochlear implant. It's the last thing they do, because it's irreversible."

Limbaugh's early perception of cochlear implants—as opposed to his current praise for the technology—is consistent with that of other recipients of neurotech therapies. Many users of neurotechnology devices have reported a similar feeling prior to deciding to go ahead with their implant: they are concerned that a cure for their particular disease or disorder is imminent and that implanting a device might interfere with that cure. Some have also felt that neurotech therapies represent a form of rehabilitation, not a cure. And many users have reported that clinicians are sometimes hesitant to recommend the procedure because of reimbursement or other financial issues. In many cases, it was difficult to even find information on neurotech therapies because the respective patient communities were often in the dark.

After receiving their devices, however, most neurotech users—including several profiled in this book--express satisfaction with their devices and many regret not opting in sooner. Even if a cure were to be found tomorrow, many still feel that it was worth the effort they expended to receive their device, recover from surgery, and undergo training.

The notion of neurotech devices as the "last resort" overshadows almost all of the technical and engineering challenges confronting the field. There's nothing wrong with the idea of searching for a drug or compound that will cure neurological diseases and disorders. But if the clinicians, manufacturers, and funding organizations supporting that strategy do so while shunning neurotech approaches that work today and will only get better in future generations, those individuals must be held accountable to the patients they have failed to help.

People living with hearing loss should not have to wait until they are unable to function and become isolated. People living with Parkinson's disease should not have to wait until they have tried all pharmaceutical options and become lethargic before considering deep brain stimulation. People with quadriplegia should not wait years to access technology to gain hand function. Obviously, there will be those who do not meet the eligibility requirements. The options of treatments should be discussed early and the risks and benefits evaluated. We should let the patient-clinician relationship be foremost in the decision-making process. Neurotechnology devices need to move from being a last resort to being an option of first discussion.

At that point, eliminating the last resort syndrome for devices, consumers won't need to have their lives fall to pieces and their quality of life plummet before they consider a neurotech device as an option.

The Trials of Trials

People with neurological diseases and disorders who choose to participate in a clinical trial of a new neurotech therapy perform a vital function for the medical device industry. But they often endure great sacrifice in doing so, and device companies, researchers, and regulators should be looking for ways to make the process less onerous and more beneficial to trial participants.

For the most part, financial risk to participants is minimized by the fact that the trial sponsor generally bears the costs associated with the device and with medical services. But as we've seen in the preceding chapters, trial participants often incur other costs, including time off from work, travel expenses, and childcare expenses.

Often trial participants are asked to sign on to a long-term contract that may affect their future plans. For example, some female participants are required to forego pregnancy as a condition of their participation.

Once enrolled in a trial, participants may not even know if they will benefit from the potential therapy. That is because most clinical trials now require a control group whose members go through all the stages of the therapy that the other members do, but for whom the device is not even turned on, or if it is, it is delivering "sham" stimulation so that investigators can see if there is a placebo effect. Generally, neither the participant nor their doctor knows whether they are in the control group or the active group until after the trial is over. Fortunately, it is becoming more common for trial sponsors to alternate participants between control and active groups, so that everybody gets an opportunity to receive the new therapy for at least part of the time.

Once a clinical trial is complete, there is no guarantee

that trial participants will get to keep their devices, even if the trial is successful and the new device is beneficial. It can be frustrating for users who have benefited from a new device to have to give it back—particularly if it is one that has been surgically implanted in their bodies. In 2009, for example, participants in a clinical trial of an implanted brain stimulation device to treat depression made by a company called Northstar Neuroscience were required to have their devices surgically explanted even though many of them got relief from their symptoms. This happened after Northstar went out of business because of a failed clinical trial for a different therapy to treat stroke. In the future, the regulatory agencies who set the rules for clinical trials will need to be more cognizant of the long-term prospects and desires of the people who participate.

Aesthetics

The pioneers who have agreed to participate in a clinical trial or who have adopted a newly approved neurotech device generally receive the first generation of a new medical product. And often, that first-generation device is not the most elegant version, since the engineers designing the product are more concerned with function than appearance. Even surgically implanted devices frequently have external components.

The typical consumer is often concerned about outward appearances such as whiter teeth, fashionable clothing, or proper hair styles. Entire industries have been built on this notion of outward appearances. For people living with neurological conditions, their desire for an acceptable outward appearance is no different. External controllers, connective wire, and surgical scars are just a few of the considerations that consumers take into account when looking at technology options. With this in mind, medical device manufacturers will need to give more thought to the outward appearance of their future customers.

Power

In our technology-driven environment, we have become more and more reliant on battery power. Look at any airport and you will find people tethered to the wall to recharge batteries of hand-held devices, laptops, and tablets. Neurotechnology is no different. Regardless of whether a neurotech device is external or surgically implanted, it generally needs power to keep it going. Many implanted neurostimulation devices contain a battery that must be recharged on a regular basis or else surgically replaced after a number of years when the battery reaches its end of life. Neurotech manufacturers are continually striving to increase the battery life of their implanted pulse generators. At the same time, they are seeking to reduce the demands on their devices by designing more efficient stimulation algorithms.

Unlike the average handheld device, when the battery dies on a neurotechnology device the user may lose a critical bodily function. It could be a function that allows the user to live independently, or fulfills a medical need, or performs a life-preserving action like breathing. Battery power is a critical component of this emerging technology and it is an area of development for a more efficient, reliable, and longer lasting battery.

Future Directions

In the years ahead, the field of neurotechnology will witness dramatic improvements as engineers develop new techniques for stimulating the nervous system and sensing neural activity. At the same time, basic research in neuroscience will undoubtedly advance our understanding of the brain and the human nervous system.

The confluence of these two disciplines, neuroscience and neural engineering, is at the heart of several new government and private initiatives to advance brain science and neurotechnology. The BRAIN initiative, announced by President Obama in 2013, has funded numerous neurotechnology research programs. Two federal agencies in particular, the National Institutes of Health (NIH) and the Defense Advanced Research Projects Administration (DARPA), have contributed tens of millions of dollars to developing new neurotech therapies for psychiatric disorders, cognitive and memory disorders, brain injuries, and spinal cord injuries. In Europe, programs like the Human Brain Project and the NEUWalk project, which funds research for neurotech therapies for treating paralysis and Parkinson's disease, will likely produce significant advances.

We can expect to see continuing improvements in the design and engineering of neurotech devices in the years ahead. We can also expect to see a wider range of diseases and disorders treated by neurotech devices. There is currently considerable effort and funding directed at developing neurotech therapies for non-neurological disorders, including obesity, heart failure, and hypertension.

While it is hard to predict exactly what the new generation of neurotech devices will look like, it is safe to say that none of them would be possible without the significant contributions of the bionic pioneers who volunteered their time and their bodies for the advancement of medical technology.

In the preceding chapters, we have offered a journey to learn the stories of people who are these pioneers. We have witnessed their struggles, their considerations, and their triumphs. Behind each one of these stories are many more individuals living with similar neurological conditions who have never been introduced to the technology. We will continue to look for new pioneers helping to expand the frontier of neurotech therapies into new areas.

Appendix: Resources

There were many neurotechnology devices featured in this book. This section provides some additional resources to learn more about the technology, clinical trials and patient advocacy organizations.

Drop Foot Stimulation for Multiple Sclerosis
Device featured: Bioness L300
www.bioness.com
Clinical Trials: Commercial device
Patient Advocacy: National MS Society, www.nationalMSsociety.org

Vagus Nerve Stimulation for Epilepsy and Seizure Management
Device featured: Cyberonics VNS Therapy,
www.cyberonics.com
Clinical Trials: Commercial device
Patient Advocacy: Epilepsy Foundation: www.epilepsy.com

Implanted Neural Prosthesis to Restore Hand Function for SCI
Device featured: Cleveland FES Center FES Hand-Grasp System,
www.fescenter.org
Clinical Trials: Yes
Patient Advocacy: National Spinal Cord Injury Association,
www.spinalcord.org

Retinal Prosthesis for Visual Impairment Resulting from Retinitis Pigmentosa
Device featured: Second Sight Argus II Retinal Prosthesis System, www.2-sight.com
Clinical Trials: Yes
Patient Advocacy: Foundation Fighting Blindness, www.blindness.org

Surface Stimulation for Upper Extremity Rehabilitation for Brain Injury
Device featured: MyndTec MyndMove,
www.myndtec.com
Clinical Trials: Commercial Device
Patient Advocacy: Internet Stroke Center,
www.strokecenter.org
Brain Injury Alliance, www.usbia.org

Sacral Nerve Stimulation for Bowel Incontinence
Device featured: Medtronic InterStim Therapy Device,
www.medtronic.com/patients/bowel-incontinence/index.htm
Clinical Trials: Commercial device
Patient Advocacy:
Patient Ambassador Program:
www.interstimambassadors.com
Video Explanation: www.youtube.com/user/MDTBowelControl
National Digestive Diseases Information Clearinghouse (NDDIC),
Fecal Incontinence Page:
www.digestive.niddk.nih.gov/ddiseases/pubs/
fecalincontinence/#info
International Foundation for Functional Gastrointestinal Disorders
(IFFGD)
www.aboutincontinence.org

Diaphragm Pacing System for ALS
Device featured: Synapse Biomedical NeuRx Diaphragm Pacing
System, www.synapsebiomedical.com
Clinical Trials: Commercial device
Patient Advocacy: ALS Association, www.alsa.org

Deep Brain Stimulation for Parkinson's Disease
Device featured: Medtronic DBS Therapy,
www.medtronicdbs.com/parkinsons/index.htm
Clinical Trials: Commercial device
Patient Advocacy: Patient Ambassador Program:
www.medtronicdbs.com/ambassador
Video Explanation: www.youtube.com/user/MedtronicDBSTherapy
National Institutes of Health Parkinson's Disease Information Pages:
www.ninds.nih.gov/disorders/parkinsons_disease/
Parkinson's Disease Foundation: www.pdf.org
National Parkinson's Foundation: www.parkinson.org

Brain Computer Interface for Communication for Locked-In Syndrome
Device featured: BrainGate2, www.braingate2.org
Clinical Trials: Yes
Patient Advocacy: American Stroke Association:
www.strokeassociation.org

Vagus Nerve Stimulation Therapy for Stroke Rehabilitation
Device featured: MicroTransponder Vivistim,
www.microtransponder.com
Clinical Trials: Yes
Patient Advocacy: National Stroke Association, www.stroke.org

About the Authors

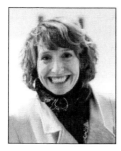

Jennifer French is the founder of Neurotech Network, a nonprofit advocacy group promoting access to new technologies for individuals with neurological disorders. She is the author of On My Feet Again (Neurotech Press, 2012).

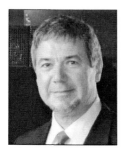

James Cavuoto is the editor and publisher of Neurotech Business Report, a newsletter covering the neurotechnology industry he founded in 2001. A biomedical engineering graduate, he has authored several research reports and articles on neurotech devices.